Targeting the IL-17 Pathway in Inflammatory Disorders

Cong-Qiu Chu

Targeting the IL-17 Pathway in Inflammatory Disorders

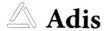

Cong-Qiu Chu
VA Portland Health Care System
Oregon Health & Science University
Portland
Oregon
USA

ISBN 978-3-319-28039-4   ISBN 978-3-319-28040-0   (eBook)
DOI 10.1007/978-3-319-28040-0

Library of Congress Control Number: 2016959037

Printed on acid-free paper

This Adis imprint is published by Springer Nature
The registered company is Springer International Publishing AG
The registered company address is Gewerbestrasse 11, 6330 Cham, Switzerland

To Hong, Max, and Owen.

Contents

Introduction

The family of interleukin-17 (IL-17), consisting of six members, is one of the most ancient host defense systems. The existence of the family was not known until 1993 when the first member, IL-17 (later renamed IL-17A), was uncovered. However, the family remained little known until 2005 when a new CD4$^+$ T-helper (Th) subset was identified. It was found that the newly described Th cells produce mainly IL-17A and IL-17F, so this new Th subset was named Th17 cells. Moreover, it was found that Th17 cells mediate many autoimmune inflammatory diseases that were previously thought to be mediated by Th1 cells. The paradigm shift of view of autoimmune inflammatory disease has had a tremendous impact on therapy of many inflammatory diseases. Highly efficacious therapy has developed by targeting the IL-17/Th17 pathway. The development of novel therapies targeting this pathway will continue for many years to come.

However, the importance of these IL-17 cytokines in host immunity against infections is not being fully appreciated. Moreover, emerging evidence indicates that activities of this family of cytokines are diverse, and antagonism between the family members has been described.

This volume will begin with a brief review of the discovery of IL-17 and their function in host defenses in the context for cautions during therapy in inflammatory diseases when IL-17 cytokine activity is blocked and then focus on the identification and regulation of Th17 cells, the role of Th17 cells in the pathogenesis of inflammatory diseases, and strategies to block IL-17 cytokine signaling and target Th17 cells for therapy of these conditions.

Abbreviations

ACR	American College of Rheumatology
Act1	NFκB activator 1 (also known as CIKS, connection to IKK and SAPK/JNK), IL-17 receptor adaptor
AD	Autosomal dominant
AIRE	Autoimmune regulator
APECED	Autoimmune polyendocrinopathy candidiasis ectodermal dystrophy
APS-1	Autoimmune polyglandular syndrome type 1
AR	Autosomal recessive
AS	Ankylosing spondylitis
BATF	Basic leucine zipper transcription factor, ATF-like
BLIMP1	B lymphocyte-induced maturation protein 1 (also known as PRDM1, PR domain zinc finger protein 1)
CARD	Caspase recruitment domain-containing protein
C/EBP	CCAAT-enhancer-binding proteins
CIA	Collagen-induced arthritis
CMC	Chronic mucocutaneous candidiasis
CNS	Central nervous system
CRP	C-reactive protein
CSF	Cerebral spinal fluid
CTLA-8	Cytotoxic T lymphocyte-associated protein 8 (it was identified as interleukin-17 [IL-17] and later renamed IL-17A)

CXC chemokines	CXC chemokines comprise a subfamily of the chemokine superfamily and are defined by the arrangement of the first two of four invariant cysteine residues found in most chemokines. In CC chemokines, these two cysteines are adjacent, while in the CXC subfamily, they are separated by a single amino acid
DC	Dendritic cells
DMARD	Disease-modifying antirheumatic drug
EAE	Experimental autoimmune encephalomyelitis
EAM	Experimental autoimmune myocarditis
EBI3	Epstein–Barr virus-induced gene 3 (a subunit of IL-27)
FOXP3	Forkhead box P3 (also known as scurfin)
GATA-3	GATA transcription factors are a family of transcription factors characterized by their ability to bind to the DNA sequence "GATA"
G-CSF	Granulocyte colony-stimulating factor
GM-CSF	Granulocyte-macrophage colony-stimulating factor
HIF1α	Hypoxia-inducible factor 1α
HLH	Helix–loop–helix
HVS	Herpesvirus saimiri
IFN	Interferon
IL	Interleukin
ILC	Innate lymphoid cell
iNKT cells	Invariant natural killer T cells
IRF4	Interferon regulatory factor 4
KC	Keratinocyte chemoattractant (also known as Groα, growth-regulated oncogene α)
LBD	Ligand-binding domain
LIX	Lipopolysaccharide-induced CXC chemokine

LTi cells	Lymphoid tissue inducer cells
MAPK	Mitogen-activated protein kinases
MCP-1	Monocyte chemoattractant protein-1
MIG	Monokine induced by gamma interferon
MIP-2	Macrophage inflammatory protein-2 (also known as CXCL2 and many other names)
MIP3α	Macrophage inflammatory protein-3α
miRNA	MicroRNA
MPO	Myeloperoxidase
MS	Multiple sclerosis
mTOR	Mammalian target of rapamycin (or mechanistic target of rapamycin; also known as FRAP1, FK506 binding protein 12-rapamycin-associated protein 1)
NFκB	Nuclear factor κB
NK cells	Natural killer cells
NO	Nitric oxide
OPC	Oropharyngeal candidiasis
OVA	Ovalbumin
PGA	Physician global assessment
PGE	Prostaglandin E
PsA	Psoriatic arthritis
PASI	Psoriasis Area Severity Index
PsO	Psoriasis
RA	Rheumatoid arthritis
RANKL	Receptor activator of nuclear factor kappa-B ligand (also known as TNFSF11, tumor necrosis factor (ligand) superfamily member 11; TRANCE, TNF-related activation-induced cytokine; OPGL, osteoprotegerin ligand; ODF, osteoclast differentiation factor)
ROR	Retinoic acid receptor (RAR)-related orphan receptor
RUNX1	Runt-related transcription factor 1 (also known as AML1, acute myeloid leukemia protein; CBFA2, core-binding factor subunit alpha-2)

SEFIR	Similar expression to fibroblast growth factor genes and IL-17R
shRNA	Short hairpin RNA
siRNA	Small interfering RNA
SNP	Single-nucleotide polymorphism
STAT	Signal transducers and activators of transcription
T-bet	T-box transcription factor (TBX21)
TCR	T cell receptor
Tfh cells	T follicular helper cells
TGF	Transforming growth factor
Th cells	T-helper cells
TIR	Toll/interleukin-1 receptor
TLR	Toll-like receptor
TNF	Tumor necrosis factor
TNFi	Tumor necrosis factor inhibitor
TNFR	Tumor necrosis factor receptor
TRAF	Tumor necrosis factor-associated factor
TYK	Tyrosine kinase

Author Biography

Cong-Qiu Chu, MD, PhD, is associate professor of medicine at Oregon Health & Science University and VA Portland Health Care System, Portland, Oregon. Dr. Chu obtained his MD from Norman Bethune University of Medical Sciences, Changchun, China, and PhD from the Kennedy Institute of Rheumatology, University of London, London, UK, and completed his internal medicine residency at Peking Union Medical College Hospital, Beijing, and Wayne State University Detroit Medical Center, Detroit, Michigan, and rheumatology fellowship at the University of Washington, Seattle. Dr. Chu has a career-long interest in the pathogenesis of rheumatoid arthritis (RA). His seminal observation that tumor necrosis factor (TNF) is overexpressed in RA joint tissue helped the development of TNF inhibitors for therapy of RA. His contribution was recognized with the European League Against Rheumatism Young Investigator Award in 1991. Dr. Chu is one of the investigators who first demonstrated that T-helper type 1 (Th1) cells are not the cell types mediating autoimmune inflammatory diseases, which were later uncovered to be mediated by Th17 cells. Dr. Chu's current research includes developing novel therapeutic strategies using RNA interference technology for precise targeting of Th17 cells for inflammatory diseases and developing optimal management strategies for early RA.

Chapter 1
Overview of IL-17 Family

1.1 Discovery and Structure of IL-17

The name of IL-17 was first proposed by Yao et al. [1] in 1995 when they discovered that an open reading frame of the T lymphotropic herpesvirus saimiri gene 13 (HSV13) exhibits 58 % homology with a previously cloned molecule, mouse cytotoxic T lymphocyte-associated protein 8 (CTLA-8) [2]. Recombinant HVS13 and CTLA-8 stimulate transcription factor NFκB activity and IL-6 secretion in fibroblasts and co-stimulate T cell proliferation. A novel cytokine receptor was also isolated and shown to bind both HVS13 and CTLA-8. Therefore, mouse CTLA-8 was named as IL-17, HVS13 as viral IL-17, and the newly cloned cytokine receptor as IL-17 receptor (IL-17R) [1]. Human IL-17 shares 72 % homology with HSV13 and 62 % with mouse IL-17 [3]. Subsequently, by homology-based cloning another 5 cytokines were identified to belong to the IL-17 gene family [4, 5, 6, 7]. The prototypic member IL-17 was renamed as IL-17A and the others as IL-17B through to F (see Table 2.1) [8].

IL-17E was found to be identical to IL-25, which was described by an independent group [9]. All IL-17 cytokines are homodimeric glycoproteins linked by a disulfide bond except IL-17B, which forms a noncovalent homodimer. All show conservation in their c-terminal region, with five spatially conserved cysteine residues accounting for a

C.-Q. Chu, *Targeting the IL-17 Pathway in Inflammatory Disorders*, DOI 10.1007/978-3-319-28040-0_1,
© Springer International Publishing Switzerland 2017

characteristic cysteine-knot formation. Of these members, IL-17A and IL-17F are most closely related and share 55 % amino acid sequences. IL-17A and IL-17F also form a heterodimer, IL-17A/F, which exerts similar functions to those of IL-17A and IL-17F (see Table 2.1) [10, 11, 12]. Homology with IL-17A for IL-17B, IL-17D, and IL-17C is in the order of 29 %, 25 %, and 23 %, respectively, and IL-17E is most distant and with only 19 % homology with IL-17A [8].

1.2   IL-17 Receptors and Signaling

IL-17 receptor (IL-17R) is also a unique cytokine receptor family [1] with five members identified to date, namely, IL-17RA, IL-17RB, IL-17RC, IL-17RD, and IL-17RE (see Table 2.1) [13]. All these IL-17 receptors contain extracellular domains composed of fibronectin type III (FnIII) domains and cytoplasmic similar expression to fibroblast growth factor (SEF) genes–IL-17R (SEFIR) domains that are loosely homologous to Toll/IL-1R domains [14, 15]. Several studies have shown that IL-17RA serves as a common receptor to mediate signals for several members of the IL-17 family (Fig. 1.1) [16, 17, 18, 19, 20, 21, 22, 23].

Indeed, the major IL-17RA interacting residues are identical among all IL-17 cytokines [24]. But IL-17RA does not bind all ligands with an equal affinity. IL-17RA has high affinity for IL-17A, about hundredfold weaker affinity for IL-17F, an intermediate affinity for IL-17A/F, and much weaker affinities for IL-17B, IL-17C, IL-17D, and IL-17E [4, 5, 16, 17, 19, 22, 25]. Interestingly, IL-17RA pairs with other IL-17Rs to form functional heterodimeric receptor complexes. This is apparently determined by the ligands, IL-17 cytokines. For example, the homodimeric IL-17A or IL-17F disfavors binding of a second molecule of IL-17RA, but selects IL-17RC to form IL-17RA-RC complex (Fig. 1.1) [24]. Similarly, other IL-17 cytokines bind their primary receptors and recruit IL-17RA to form a functional heterodimeric receptor complex. IL-17A and IL-17F and IL-17A/F bind to

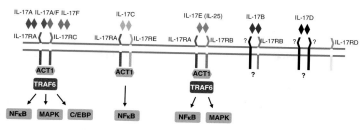

FIGURE 1.1 IL-17 receptors. The IL-17R family comprises five members: IL-17RA, IL-17RB, IL-17RC, IL-17RD, and IL-17RE. IL-17RA is a common receptor that forms heterodimers with other IL-17Rs for ligand binding and signal transduction: IL-17RA-RC for IL-17A, IL-17F, and IL-17A/F; IL-17RA-RE for IL-17C; IL-17RA-RB for IL-17E (IL-25). It is not clear whether IL-17RB also forms a homodimer for IL-17B; IL-17RD remains an orphan receptor, but it regulates IL-17A signaling and forms TNFR2–IL-17RD receptor complex. The receptor for IL-17D has not been identified. IL-17RA-RC, IL-17RA-RB, and IL-17RA-RE transduce signal via adaptor molecule Act1. *Act1* NFκB activator 1 (also known as *CIKS* connection to IKK and SAPK/JNK), *IL-17RA* IL-17 receptor adaptor, *C/EBPs* CCAAT-enhancer-binding proteins, *MAPKs* mitogen-activated protein kinases, *NFκB* nuclear factor κB, *TRAF* tumor necrosis factor-associated factor

receptor complex IL-17RA-RC, IL-17C to IL-17RA-RE, and IL-17E (IL-25) to IL-17RA-RB (Fig. 1.1) [13]. The redundant activities of IL-17A and IL-17F are partially attributed to their binding to the same IL-17RA-RC receptor complex, and yet the distinct activities of the two cytokines may be due to the different binding affinities to the receptor complex [26]. Both components of the heterodimeric receptor complex are required for signaling. For instance, deficiency of either IL-17RA or IL-17RC can completely abolish the inflammatory function of IL-17A and IL-17F [12, 21, 27, 28].

The proinflammatory and host defense effects of IL-17A and IL-17F are executed chiefly by activation of NFκB and MAPK pathways. A signal from IL-17R is first relayed by a cytosolic protein, signaling adaptor, called Act1 (NFκB activator 1, also known as CIKS) (Fig. 1.2) [29].

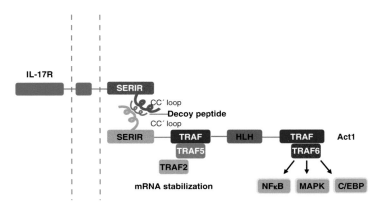

FIGURE 1.2 Structure of Act1. Act1 is IL-17R adaptor which relays IL-17 cytokine–IL-17R signaling. It contains a SEFIR domain that binds cytoplasmic SEFIR domain of IL-17Rs. A decoy peptide correspondence of the sequence of CC' loop of Act1 SEFIR domain can block the IL-17A and IL-17E (IL-25) signaling, indicating interruption of interaction between Act1 and IL-17R is potentially therapeutic. *C/EBP* CCAAT-enhancer-binding proteins, *HLH* helix–loop–helix, *MAPKs* mitogen-activated protein kinases, *NFκB* nuclear factor κB, *SEFIR* similar expression to fibroblast growth factor genes and IL-17R, *TRAF* tumor necrosis factor-associated factor

Act1 is essential for IL-17 signal transduction. Deficiency of Act1 results in a loss of IL-17-dependent NFκB activation and proinflammatory cytokine production [29, 30]. Upon ligand stimulation of IL-17R, Act1 is recruited to the IL-17R complex. Act1 also contains a SEFIR domain, which binds to the SEFIR region of IL-17R through homotypic interactions [13, 31]. The activated Act1 then binds tumor necrosis factor-associated factor (TRAF)-6 via a TRAF binding domains of Act1 (Figs. 1.1 and 1.2). TRAF6 mediates further downstream cascade interactions to lead to activation of NFκB, MAPK, and C/EBP pathways and the activation of target genes [13].

The importance of Act1 in autoimmunity and inflammatory diseases has been demonstrated in animal models of inflammatory diseases. For instance, mice with deficiency of

Act1 have reduced demyelination in a cuprizone-induced multiple sclerosis (MS) model, which is known to be mediated by IL-17 signaling [32]. Act1-deficient mice are protected from collagen-induced arthritis (CIA) [33]. These data suggest that Act1 is a candidate target for therapeutic intervention in human inflammatory diseases.

As in other cytokine signaling, IL-17/IL-17R signaling is also finely regulated. Many regulators have been described to involve positive and negative regulation of the IL-17/IL-17R signaling pathway at various stages [13]. Modulation of these regulatory factors is potentially of therapeutic benefit. Soluble IL-17RA, IL-17RB, and IL-17RC naturally exist and may function as decoy receptor to regulate IL-17–IL-17R signaling in vivo. Indeed, fused with immunoglobulin G (IgG) Fc fragment, soluble IL-17RA (IL-17RA-Fc) is able to suppress IL-17A signaling in cultured cells; IL-17RC-Fc suppresses the effect of IL-17A and IL-17F [27], and IL-17RB-Fc is able to block IL-17E signaling [34]. These soluble receptor-Fc fusion proteins are highly likely to be evaluated as therapeutic agents (Fig. 5.1b).

Signaling through the IL-17R complex can influence function of other IL-17 cytokines. Chang et al. [17] observed that IL-17C is highly expressed in the central nervous system of mice with experimental autoimmune encephalomyelitis (EAE). IL-17C knockout mice exhibited a striking reduction of incidence and severity of EAE along with reduction of Th17 cells [17]. IL-17C signaling through IL-17RA-RE [17, 18, 19] further increases IL-17RE expression on Th17 cells and increases IL-17A, IL-17F, and IL-22 production. Skin keratinocytes and intestine epithelial cells constitutively express IL-17RE and can respond to IL-17C [18, 19]. These findings indicate that IL-17C may be another target for therapy in Th17-mediated inflammatory diseases, but caution needs to be taken for its protective effect in intestines.

It is noteworthy that IL-17RD remains an orphan receptor, i.e., no ligand has been identified to bind IL-17RD. Interestingly, IL-17RD is able to critically regulate the activities of IL-17A [23, 35]. IL-17RD deficiency abolished

IL-17A-induced neutrophil recruitment, which is correlated with reduced p38 MARP kinase and expression of the neutrophil chemokine MIP-2. On the other hand, IL-17RD deficiency results in enhanced IL-17A induced activation of NFκB and IL-6 and keratinocyte chemoattractant expression. This negative regulation is through IL-17RD disruption of the interaction of Act1 and TRAF6 [23, 35].

Recent studies also revealed that IL-17RD negatively regulates TLR response [36]. IL-17RD deficiency leads to increased susceptibility to TLR-induced septic shock because of enhanced proinflammatory signaling. The suppressive effect of IL-17RD is via interaction of SEFIR domain of IL-17RD with Toll/interleukin-1 receptor (TIR) domain of TLR [36]. Moreover, IL-17RD can form a heterodimer with TNFR2 to activate NFκB [37]. These data indicate a complex regulatory mechanism that IL-17RD is involved with other inflammatory pathways.

References

1. Yao Z, Fanslow WC, Seldin MF, et al. Herpesvirus Saimiri encodes a new cytokine, IL-17, which binds to a novel cytokine receptor. Immunity. 1995;3:811–21.
2. Rouvier E, Luciani MF, Mattei MG, Denizot F, Golstein P. CTLA-8, cloned from an activated T cell, bearing AU-rich messenger RNA instability sequences, and homologous to a herpesvirus saimiri gene. J Immunol. 1993;150:5445–56.
3. Yao Z, Painter SL, Fanslow WC, et al. Human IL-17: a novel cytokine derived from T cells. J Immunol. 1995;155:5483–6.
4. Lee J, Ho WH, Maruoka M, et al. IL-17E, a novel proinflammatory ligand for the IL-17 receptor homolog IL-17Rh1. J Biol Chem. 2001;276:1660–4.
5. Li H, Chen J, Huang A, et al. Cloning and characterization of IL-17B and IL-17C, two new members of the IL-17 cytokine family. Proc Natl Acad Sci U S A. 2000;97:773–8.
6. Starnes T, Broxmeyer HE, Robertson MJ, Hromas R. Cutting edge: IL-17D, a novel member of the IL-17 family, stimulates cytokine production and inhibits hemopoiesis. J Immunol. 2002; 169:642–6.

7. Starnes T, Robertson MJ, Sledge G, et al. Cutting edge: IL-17F, a novel cytokine selectively expressed in activated T cells and monocytes, regulates angiogenesis and endothelial cell cytokine production. J Immunol. 2001;167:4137–40.

8. Kolls JK, Linden A. Interleukin-17 family members and inflammation. Immunity. 2004;21:467–76.

9. Fort MM, Cheung J, Yen D, et al. IL-25 induces IL-4, IL-5, and IL-13 and Th2-associated pathologies in vivo. Immunity. 2001;15:985–95.

10. Chang SH, Dong C. A novel heterodimeric cytokine consisting of IL-17 and IL-17F regulates inflammatory responses. Cell Res. 2007;17:435–40.

11. Wright JF, Guo Y, Quazi A, et al. Identification of an interleukin 17F/17A heterodimer in activated human CD4+ T cells. J Biol Chem. 2007;282:13447–55.

12. Wright JF, Bennett F, Li B, et al. The human IL-17F/IL-17A heterodimeric cytokine signals through the IL-17RA/IL-17RC receptor complex. J Immunol. 2008;181:2799–805.

13. Gu C, Wu L, Li X. IL-17 family: cytokines, receptors and signaling. Cytokine. 2013;64:477–85.

14. Novatchkova M, Leibbrandt A, Werzowa J, Neubuser A, Eisenhaber F. The STIR-domain superfamily in signal transduction, development and immunity. Trends Biochem Sci. 2003;28:226–9.

15. Kramer JM, Hanel W, Shen F, et al. Cutting edge: identification of a pre-ligand assembly domain (PLAD) and ligand binding site in the IL-17 receptor. J Immunol. 2007;179:6379–83.

16. Ely LK, Fischer S, Garcia KC. Structural basis of receptor sharing by interleukin 17 cytokines. Nat Immunol. 2009;10:1245–51.

17. Chang SH, Reynolds JM, Pappu BP, et al. Interleukin-17C promotes Th17 cell responses and autoimmune disease via interleukin-17 receptor E. Immunity. 2011;35:611–21.

18. Song X, Zhu S, Shi P, et al. IL-17RE is the functional receptor for IL-17C and mediates mucosal immunity to infection with intestinal pathogens. Nat Immunol. 2011;12:1151–8.

19. Ramirez-Carrozzi V, Sambandam A, Luis E, et al. IL-17C regulates the innate immune function of epithelial cells in an autocrine manner. Nat Immunol. 2011;12:1159–66.

20. Ho AW, Shen F, Conti HR, et al. IL-17RC is required for immune signaling via an extended SEF/IL-17R signaling domain in the cytoplasmic tail. J Immunol. 2010;185:1063–70.

21. Toy D, Kugler D, Wolfson M, et al. Cutting edge: interleukin 17 signals through a heteromeric receptor complex. J Immunol. 2006;177:36–9.
22. Rickel EA, Siegel LA, Yoon BR, et al. Identification of functional roles for both IL-17RB and IL-17RA in mediating IL-25-induced activities. J Immunol. 2008;181:4299–310.
23. Rong Z, Wang A, Li Z, et al. IL-17RD (Sef or IL-17RLM) interacts with IL-17 receptor and mediates IL-17 signaling. Cell Res. 2009;19:208–15.
24. Liu S, Song X, Chrunyk BA, et al. Crystal structures of interleukin 17 A and its complex with IL-17 receptor A. Nat Commun. 2013;4:1888.
25. Shi Y, Ullrich SJ, Zhang J, et al. A novel cytokine receptor-ligand pair. Identification, molecular characterization, and in vivo immunomodulatory activity. J Biol Chem. 2000;275:19167–76.
26. Jin W, Dong C. IL-17 cytokines in immunity and inflammation. Emerg Microbes Infect 2013;2:e60.
27. Kuestner RE, Taft DW, Haran A, et al. Identification of the IL-17 receptor related molecule IL-17RC as the receptor for IL-17F. J Immunol. 2007;179:5462–73.
28. Chang SH, Dong C. Signaling of interleukin-17 family cytokines in immunity and inflammation. Cell Signal. 2011;23:1069–75.
29. Chang SH, Park H, Dong C. Act1 adaptor protein is an immediate and essential signaling component of interleukin-17 receptor. J Biol Chem. 2006;281:35603–7.
30. Qian Y, Liu C, Hartupee J, et al. The adaptor Act1 is required for interleukin 17-dependent signaling associated with autoimmune and inflammatory disease. Nat Immunol. 2007;8:247–56.
31. Song X, Qian Y. IL-17 family cytokines mediated signaling in the pathogenesis of inflammatory diseases. Cell Signal. 2013;25:2335–47.
32. Kang Z, Liu L, Spangler R, et al. IL-17-induced Act1-mediated signaling is critical for cuprizone-induced demyelination. J Neurosci. 2012;32:8284–92.
33. Pisitkun P, Claudio E, Ren N, Wang H, Siebenlist U. The adaptor protein CIKS/ACT1 is necessary for collagen-induced arthritis, and it contributes to the production of collagen-specific antibody. Arthritis Rheum. 2010;62:3334–44.
34. Wang YH, Angkasekwinai P, Lu N, et al. IL-25 augments type 2 immune responses by enhancing the expansion and functions of TSLP-DC-activated Th2 memory cells. J Exp Med. 2007;204:1837–47.

35. Mellett M, Atzei P, Horgan A, et al. Orphan receptor IL-17RD tunes IL-17A signalling and is required for neutrophilia. Nat Commun. 2012;3:1119.
36. Mellett M, Atzei P, Bergin R, et al. Orphan receptor IL-17RD regulates Toll-like receptor signalling via SEFIR/TIR interactions. Nat Commun. 2015;6:6669.
37. Yang S, Wang Y, Mei K, et al. Tumor necrosis factor receptor 2 (TNFR2).interleukin-17 receptor D (IL-17RD) heteromerization reveals a novel mechanism for NF-kappaB activation. J Biol Chem. 2015;290:861–71.

Chapter 2
IL-17 in Host Defense

2.1 Cellular Source of IL-17

Many cell types including immune and nonimmune cells are able to produce IL-17 cytokines for host defense. In particular, innate immune cells such as γδT cells [1]. Recent studies indicate that γδT cells are the major initial IL-17 producers in acute infections [2]. Some γδT cells have IL-17-producing capacities without explicit induction of an immune response. These γδT cells preferentially reside in the skin and mucosal membranes [2]. Other innate immune cells producing IL-17 include NK, iNKT, mast cells, lymph tissue inducer (LTi) cells, group 3 innate lymphoid cells (ILC3) [3], and macrophages. Adoptive immune cells producing IL-17 include Th17 cells and Tc17 cells. Nonimmune cells include epithelial cells and keratinocytes, which are more likely for host defense. Adoptive immune cells producing IL-17 include Th17 cells and Tc17 cells. While CD8+ Tc17 cells are more likely to participate in host defense, CD4+ Th17 cells are more likely to participate in chronic inflammation in inflammatory diseases. ILC3 cells are found in the lung, gut, and skin. Currently, IL-17-producing ILC3 cells are often associated with inflammation [3–5], but their physiological property in host defense is not fully appreciated (Table 2.1) [6].

Many cell types express IL-17 receptors indicating the wide range of effects that IL-17 cytokines can take place to

C.-Q. Chu, *Targeting the IL-17 Pathway in Inflammatory Disorders*, DOI 10.1007/978-3-319-28040-0_2,
© Springer International Publishing Switzerland 2017

TABLE 2.1 Cellular source of IL-17 cytokines and their major functions

IL-17 cytokine	Cellular source	Receptors	Main function in host defense
IL-17A (IL-17)	γδT, iNKT, LTi, ILC3, Th17, Tc17, mast cells, keratinocytes, macrophages	IL-17RA-RC	Host defense against extracellular bacterial and fungal infections
IL-17F	γδT, iNKT, LTi, ILC3, Th17, Tc17, mast cells, keratinocytes, macrophages	IL-17RA-RC	Host defense against extracellular bacterial and fungal infections
IL-17A/F	From the same cells as IL-17A or IL-17F	IL-17RA-RC	Similar to IL-17A or IL-17F
IL-17B	Chondrocytes, intestinal epithelial cells, neurons, and breast cancer cells	IL-17RB-?	Bacterial infection
IL-17C	Endothelial cells and leukocytes	IL-17RA-RE	Cooperates with Th17 cells in bacterial infections; promotes Th17 cells via IL-17RE signaling
IL-17D	Skeletal muscle, brain, adipose tissue, heart, lung, and pancreas	?	Tumor rejection
IL-17E (IL-25)	Epithelial cells	IL-17RA-RB	Helminth infections via induction of Th2 cells
		IL-17RD (orphan receptor)	Negatively regulates TLR response, positively regulates IL-17A-mediated neutrophil recruitment, and downregulates IL-17A-mediated NFκB activation, forming TNFR2–IL-17RD receptor complex to activate NFκB

ILC innate lymphoid cell, *iNKT cells* invariant natural killer T cells, *LTi cells* lymphoid tissue inducer cells, *NFκB* nuclear factor κB, *TNFR* tumor necrosis factor receptor

influence cell biology. The major physiological function of IL-17 is mediating host mucosal defense against extracellular bacterial and fungal infection. This function is mainly achieved via induction of local tissue inflammation as a result from cooperation of IL-17 with other cytokines and mediators.

2.2   Induction of Chemokines and Inflammatory Cytokines by IL-17

The major feature of IL-17 signal-deficient mice is the reduced number of neutrophils at the site of inflammation, which indicates the critical role of IL-17 in recruiting neutrophils. IL-17RA knockout mice which were challenged with *Klebsiella pneumoniae* displayed a significant reduction of neutrophils in the infected lungs with 100 % mortality [7]. The reduced accumulation of neutrophils in the infection sites is associated with decreased expression of granulocyte colony-stimulating factor (G-CSF) and MIP-2 in the lung [7]. Inversely, ectopic expression of IL-17 resulted in a strong neutrophilic response [8]. However, IL-17 does not affect function of neutrophils. Neutrophils from IL-17RA-deficient mice are intrinsically normal as they migrate normally in response to attractants and produce normal levels of MPO [9]. Subsequent in vitro studies have demonstrated that IL-17A induces expression of CXC chemokines by epithelial cells (Table 2.2) and other cell types. Many CXC chemokines are induced by IL-17A. The key chemokines in mice are CXCL1 and CXCL5 [10], while IL-8 (CXCL8) in humans [11] are the most neutrophil-attracting molecules induced by IL-17A. These data indicate that IL-17A indirectly act on neutrophils.

IL-17A-induced inflammation is also via induction of other pro-inflammatory cytokines. As shown in Table 2.2, several studies demonstrated that IL-17A is a potent inducer of IL-6 production by several cell types. IL-6 is a potent stimulator for Th17 cell differentiation suggesting a positive feedback mechanism induced by IL-17A [12]. Other inflammatory cytokines induced by IL-17A include tumor necrosis

TABLE 2.2 IL-17-induced expression of molecules involved in innate immunity

Molecules induced by IL-17	Cell types	References
Chemokines		
CXCL1 (KC, Groα)	Lung, bronchial epithelial cells, osteoblasts (synergy with TNF), mesothelial cells, intestinal epithelial cells, fibroblasts	[10, 12–17]
CXCL2 (MIP2)	Lung, osteoblasts (synergy with TNF)	[7, 10]
CXCL5 (LIX, GCP2)	Osteoblasts (synergy with TNF)	[10]
CXCL8 (IL-8)	Fibroblasts, endothelial cells, bronchial epithelial cells, renal epithelial cells	[11, 13, 16, 18–21]
CXCL9 (MIG)	Lung	[22]
CXCL10 (IP10)	Lung	[22]
CXCL11	Lung	[22]
CCL2 (MCP-1)	Osteoblasts (synergy with TNF), renal epithelial cells, intestinal epithelial cells	[10, 14, 20]
CCL20 (MIP3α)	Bronchial epithelial cells	[23]
Cytokines		
IL-6	Fibroblasts, endothelial cells, bronchial epithelial cells, kidney epithelial cells' renal epithelial cells, macrophages	[11, 12, 18, 20, 21, 24–27]
IL-1β	Macrophages	[25]
TNF-α	Fibroblasts, macrophages	[25, 26]
G-CSF	Lung, fibroblasts	[7, 11, 27, 28]
GM-CSF	Fibroblasts, bronchial epithelial cells, endothelial cells	[11, 28, 29]
IL-17A	Fibroblasts	[26]

(continued)

TABLE 2.2 (continued)

Molecules induced by IL-17	Cell types	References
Acute-phase proteins		
CRP	Hepatocytes	[30]
Lipocalin 2 (24p3)	Osteoblasts, fibroblasts	[31, 32]
Antimicrobial peptides		
β-Defensins	Bronchial epithelial cells	[33]
Mucins	Bronchial epithelial cells	[34]
Calgranulins (S100 proteins)	Keratinocytes	[35]

Adapted from © Elsevier, Table 2 in [36]. All rights reserved. Gaffen et al. [36]

CRP C-reactive protein, *G-CSF* granulocyte colony-stimulating factor, *GM-CSF* granulocyte-macrophage colony-stimulating factor, *IP-10* interferon-γ-inducible protein 10

factor (TNF), IL-1β, and granulocyte-macrophage colony-stimulating factor (GM-CSF) [25, 26]. IL-17 synergizes with TNF and IL-1β in induction of CXC chemokine expression [13, 14, 19]. IL-17 is also a potent inducer for NO synthase and cyclooxygenase expression and leads to an increase in nitric oxide (NO) and prostaglandin E2 (PGE2) production in various cell types, and this process is synergized by TNF and IL-1β [37, 38].

In addition, IL-17A contributes to host defense via promotion of antimicrobial peptides. IL-17A regulates expression of several antimicrobial molecules including β-defensins, calgranulins (S100 proteins), and mucins [33–35, 39]. Defensins acting as natural antibiotics are potent antimicrobial peptides for host defense in the lung, skin, and gut [40, 41].

Systemically, IL-17A promotes expression of acute-phase protein lipocalin 2 [31, 32]. Lipocalin 2 binds to bacterial siderophores. Siderophores are iron-scavenging molecules that are necessary for the survival of bacteria and fungi. Lipocalin 2 binds siderophores and therefore inhibits the iron uptake by bacteria in the body [42]. It has been shown that lipocalin 2 is required for pulmonary defense against *Klebsiella* infection [43] and *Escherichia coli* in the intestine [42].

2.3   Importance of IL-17 Cytokines in Mucosal and Cutaneous Immunity in Host Defense

The importance of IL-17 cytokines in mucosal and cutaneous immunity in host defense was first indicated by a series of experiments in IL-17RA- or IL-17A-deficient mice [7, 44, 45]. Mice deficient in IL-17RA are highly susceptible to *Klebsiella pneumoniae* infection with a greater than 50 % fatality [7]. This is correlated with markedly decreased recruitment of neutrophils to the airway. Oropharyngeal candidiasis (OPC) is severe in IL-23- and IL-17RA-deficient mice, whereas IL-12-deficient mice showed low fungal burden and no overt infection [44]. This finding clearly indicates the critical role of IL-17A in mucosal immunity against *Candida* infection and that the IL-12 and Th1 pathway is less important. Furthermore, the source of IL-17A for this immunity is identified as γδT cells and Th17 cells [46]. Mice deficient in γδT cells develop exacerbations of skin *Staphylococcus aureus* infection with severely impaired neutrophil recruitment. This phenotype is similar to IL-17RA-deficient mice. Interestingly, a single dose of IL-17A could restore the impaired immunity in γδT cell deficiency. These data clearly define a critical role of IL-17A in skin defense against *Staphylococcus aureus* infection and the importance of the cellular source of IL-17A being the epidermal γδT cells [45].

The protective role of IL-17 cytokines in host defense in humans is categorically demonstrated in patients with genetic defect in pathways leading to defective production of IL-17 (Table 2.3). The disease severity in patients with gene mutations varies from mild focal infection to systemic and fatal

Table 2.3 Genetic defects affecting the Th17/IL-17 pathway

Gene	Mutation/inheritance	Protein function affected	Immunodeficiency	Clinical phenotype and infection	Ref
Mutations affecting IL-17–IL-17R binding					
Il17f	IL-17F-S65L/AD	Impaired IL-17F and IL-17A/F binding to IL-17RA	↓ fibroblast production of GROα and IL-6	CMC C. albicans S. aureus	[51]
Il17ra	IL-17RA-Q284X/AR	Lack of IL-17RA extracellular domain	Loss of binding of IL-17A, IL-17F, and IL-17A/F on fibroblasts and leukocytes; ↓ GROa and IL-6 production	CMC C. albicans S. aureus	[51]
Il-17rc	IL-17RC-Q138X, R378X, R378X/AR	Lack of IL-17RC extracellular domain	Loss of binding of IL-17A, IL-17F, and IL-17A/F on fibroblasts ↓ GROa and IL-6 production	CMC C. albicans	[52]

(continued)

TABLE 2.3 (continued)

Gene	Mutation/inheritance	Protein function affected	Immunodeficiency	Clinical phenotype and infection	Ref
Mutations affecting IL-17 signaling					
Act1	ACT1 – T536I/AR	Impaired interaction with IL-17R	Impaired IL-17A and IL-17F signaling	CMC C. albicans	[53]
Mutations affecting Th17 cells					
Rorc	ROR-γ-S38L, Q329X, Q441X ROR-γt-S17L, Q308X, Q420X/AR	Impaired binding to IL-17A gene	Impaired Th17 cell differentiation, ↓ IL-17A and IL-17F production by innate immune cells, decreased size of thymus, lack of some lymph nodes, impaired IFN-γ production	C. albicans Mycobacteria	[54]

Stat3	STAT3 >20 mutations/AD	Impaired DNA binding or SH2 domain or AT	Impaired Th17 cell differentiation, ↓ production of IL-17A and IL-17F by unconventional T cells	Hyper-IgE (Job's) syndrome: *S. aureus*	[55–61]
Stat1	STAT1 >30 mutations/AR	Gain-of-function: coiled-coil domain with increased STAT-1 phosphorylation	Impaired Th17 cell differentiation, production of autoantibodies to IL-17F	CMC *C. albicans*	[62–64]
Card9	CARD9-15 mutations/AR	CARD	Impaired Th17 cell differentiation, impaired neutrophil killing	Mucocutaneous candidiasis, systemic fungal infections	[65]
Dectin1	DECTIN-1-Y238X/ AD	Impaired β-glucan binding	Th17 cell differentiation, ↓ IL-6 and TNF production	Mucocutaneous candidiasis	[66, 67]

(continued)

TABLE 2.3 (continued)

Gene	Mutation/inheritance	Protein function affected	Immunodeficiency	Clinical phenotype and infection	Ref
Tyk2	TYK-2 – C70HfsX21, L767X, T1106HfsX4, E154X, S50HfsX1, R638X/AR	Truncated protein	Impaired response to IL-23, IL-6, IL-12, and IFN-α/β ↓ IL-17A and IL-17F production in vitro	Mycobacteria 1 patient has hyper-IgE phenotype	[68]
Il2b	IL-12B (p40) – 9 mutations/AR	Impaired binding to IL-12R	Impaired Th1 and Th17 cell differentiation	Mycobacteria, *Candida, Klebsiella, Nocardia, Salmonella*	[69]
Il-12rb1	IL-12RB1 - > 100 mutations/AR	Signal transduction	Impaired Th1 and Th17 cell differentiation	Mycobacteria, *Candida, Klebsiella, Nocardia, Salmonella*	[55, 70, 71]

Mutations promoting autoantibodies to IL-17

Aire	AR ~100 mutations AD – G228W	Impaired DNA binding and/or multimerization domain SAND	Production of autoantibodies to IL-17a, IL-17F, and IL-22	CMC, APS-1/ APECED *C. albicans* *S. aureus*	[47–50]

Adapted from © Elsevier, Table 1 in [72]

Act1 NFκB activator 1 (also known as *CIKS* connection to IKK and SAPK/JNK), IL-17 receptor adaptor, *AD* autosomal dominant, *AIRE* autoimmune regulator, *APECED* autoimmune polyendocrinopathy-candidiasis-ectodermal dystrophy, *APS-1* autoimmune polyglandular syndrome type 1, *AR* autosomal recessive, *CARD* caspase recruitment domain-containing protein, *CMC* chronic mucocutaneous candidiasis, *ROR* retinoic acid receptor (RAR)-related orphan receptor, *STAT* signal transducers and activators of transcription, *TYK* tyrosine kinase

conditions. In the context of blockade of the IL-17 pathway for therapy, perhaps the phenotype in patients with *Aire* deficiency more closely mimics the therapeutic blockade of IL-17 signaling. Indeed, patients with *Aire* deficiency produce auto-antibodies against IL-17A, IL-17F, and IL-22 [47–50].

Results from a recent mouse model of OPC provide useful information for interpreting clinical findings when IL-17 cytokines or components in IL-17 signaling pathway are inhibited. The study demonstrates a hierarchy as to the degree of susceptibility to OPC in the setting of antibody therapy, in the order of severity of *Candida albicans* infection: anti-IL-17A plus anti-IL-17F antibodies > anti-IL-17A or anti-IL-17RA antibodies [73].

IL-17 cytokines are also important in immunity against systemic fungal infection [74, 75]. IL-17RA-deficient mice rapidly succumbed to systemic infection of *Candida albicans* [74]. IL-17RA deficiency has a profound impairment in NK cell dysfunction with decreased GM-CSF production by NK cells [75].

References

1. Hirota K, Ahlfors H, Duarte JH, Stockinger B. Regulation and function of innate and adaptive interleukin-17-producing cells. EMBO Rep. 2012;13:113–20.
2. Chien YH, Meyer C, Bonneville M. Gammadelta T cells: first line of defense and beyond. Annu Rev Immunol. 2014;32:121–55.
3. Kim HY, Lee HJ, Chang YJ, et al. Interleukin-17-producing innate lymphoid cells and the NLRP3 inflammasome facilitate obesity-associated airway hyperreactivity. Nat Med. 2014;20:54–61.
4. Dyring-Andersen B, Geisler C, Agerbeck C, et al. Increased number and frequency of group 3 innate lymphoid cells in nonlesional psoriatic skin. Br J Dermatol. 2014;170:609–16.
5. Song C, Lee JS, Gilfillan S, et al. Unique and redundant functions of NKp46+ ILC3s in models of intestinal inflammation. J Exp Med. 2015;212:1869–82.

6. Montaldo E, Juelke K, Romagnani C. Group 3 innate lymphoid cells (ILC3s): Origin, differentiation, and plasticity in humans and mice. Eur J Immunol. 2015;45:2171–82.
7. Ye P, Rodriguez FH, Kanaly S, et al. Requirement of interleukin 17 receptor signaling for lung CXC chemokine and granulocyte colony-stimulating factor expression, neutrophil recruitment, and host defense. J Exp Med. 2001;194:519–27.
8. Schwarzenberger P, La Russa V, Miller A, et al. Kolls, IL-17 stimulates granulopoiesis in mice: use of an alternate, novel gene therapy-derived method for in vivo evaluation of cytokines. J Immunol. 1998;161:6383–9.
9. Yu JJ, Ruddy MJ, Wong GC, et al. An essential role for IL-17 in preventing pathogen-initiated bone destruction: recruitment of neutrophils to inflamed bone requires IL-17 receptor-dependent signals. Blood. 2007;109:3794–802.
10. Ruddy MJ, Shen F, Smith JB, Sharma A, Gaffen SL. Interleukin-17 regulates expression of the CXC chemokine LIX/CXCL5 in osteoblasts: implications for inflammation and neutrophil recruitment. J Leukoc Biol. 2004;76:135–44.
11. Fossiez F, Djossou O, Chomarat P, et al. T cell interleukin-17 induces stromal cells to produce proinflammatory and hemato-poietic cytokines. J Exp Med. 1996;183:2593–603.
12. Ogura H, Murakami M, Okuyama Y, et al. Interleukin-17 pro-motes autoimmunity by triggering a positive-feedback loop via interleukin-6 induction. Immunity. 2008;29:628–36.
13. Jones CE, Chan K. Interleukin-17 stimulates the expression of interleukin-8, growth-related oncogene-alpha, and granulocyte-colony-stimulating factor by human airway epithelial cells. Am J Respir Cell Mol Biol. 2002;26:748–53.
14. Awane M, Andres PG, Li DJ, Reinecker HC. NF-kappa B-inducing kinase is a common mediator of IL-17-, TNF-alpha-, and IL-1 beta-induced chemokine promoter activation in intes-tinal epithelial cells. J Immunol. 1999;162:5337–44.
15. Aujla SJ, Chan YR, Zheng M, et al. IL-22 mediates mucosal host defense against Gram-negative bacterial pneumonia. Nat Med. 2008;14:275–81.
16. Prause O, Laan M, Lotvall J, Linden A. Pharmacological modu-lation of interleukin-17-induced GCP-2-, GRO-alpha- and inter-leukin-8 release in human bronchial epithelial cells. Eur J Pharmacol. 2003;462:193–8.
17. Witowski J, Pawlaczyk K, Breborowicz A, et al. IL-17 stimulates intraperitoneal neutrophil infiltration through the release of

GRO alpha chemokine from mesothelial cells. J Immunol. 2000;165:5814–21.

18. Yao Z, Painter SL, Fanslow WC, et al. Human IL-17: a novel cytokine derived from T cells. J Immunol. 1995;155:5483–6.

19. Laan M, Cui ZH, Hoshino H, et al. Neutrophil recruitment by human IL-17 via C-X-C chemokine release in the airways. J Immunol. 1999;162:2347–52.

20. Van Kooten C, Boonstra JG, Paape ME, et al. Interleukin-17 activates human renal epithelial cells in vitro and is expressed during renal allograft rejection. J Am Soc Nephrol. 1998;9:1526–34.

21. Laan M, Lotvall J, Chung KF, Linden A. IL-17-induced cytokine release in human bronchial epithelial cells in vitro: role of mitogen-activated protein (MAP) kinases. Br J Pharmacol. 2001;133:200–6.

22. Khader SA, Bell GK, Pearl JE, et al. IL-23 and IL-17 in the establishment of protective pulmonary CD4+ T cell responses after vaccination and during Mycobacterium tuberculosis challenge. Nat Immunol. 2007;8:369–77.

23. Kao CY, Huang F, Chen Y, et al. Up-regulation of CC chemokine ligand 20 expression in human airway epithelium by IL-17 through a JAK-independent but MEK/NF-kappaB-dependent signaling pathway. J Immunol. 2005;175:6676–85.

24. Yao Z, Fanslow WC, Seldin MF, et al. Herpesvirus Saimiri encodes a new cytokine, IL-17, which binds to a novel cytokine receptor. Immunity. 1995;3:811–21.

25. Jovanovic DV, Di Battista JA, Martel-Pelletier J, et al. IL-17 stimulates the production and expression of proinflammatory cytokines, IL-beta and TNF-alpha, by human macrophages. J Immunol. 1998;160:3513–21.

26. van Hamburg JP, Asmawidjaja PS, Davelaar N, et al. Th17 cells, but not Th1 cells, from patients with early rheumatoid arthritis are potent inducers of matrix metalloproteinases and proinflammatory cytokines upon synovial fibroblast interaction, including autocrine interleukin-17 A production. Arthritis Rheum. 2011;63:73–83.

27. Cai XY, Gommoll Jr CP, Justice L, Narula SK, Fine JS. Regulation of granulocyte colony-stimulating factor gene expression by interleukin-17. Immunol Lett. 1998;62:51–8.

28. Andoh A, Yasui H, Inatomi O, et al. Interleukin-17 augments tumor necrosis factor-alpha-induced granulocyte and granulocyte/macrophage colony-stimulating factor release from human colonic myofibroblasts. J Gastroenterol. 2005;40:802–10.

29. Laan M, Prause O, Miyamoto M, et al. A role of GM-CSF in the accumulation of neutrophils in the airways caused by IL-17 and TNF-alpha. Eur Respir J. 2003;21:387–93.

30. Patel DN, King CA, Bailey SR, et al. Interleukin-17 stimulates C-reactive protein expression in hepatocytes and smooth muscle cells via p38 MAPK and ERK1/2-dependent NF-kappaB and C/EBPbeta activation. J Biol Chem. 2007;282:27229–38.

31. Shen F, Hu Z, Goswami J, Gaffen SL. Identification of common transcriptional regulatory elements in interleukin-17 target genes. J Biol Chem. 2006;281:24138–48.

32. Shen F, Ruddy MJ, Plamondon P, Gaffen SL. Cytokines link osteoblasts and inflammation: microarray analysis of interleukin-17- and TNF-alpha-induced genes in bone cells. J Leukoc Biol. 2005;77:388–99.

33. Kao CY, Chen Y, Thai P, et al. IL-17 markedly up-regulates beta-defensin-2 expression in human airway epithelium via JAK and NF-kappaB signaling pathways. J Immunol. 2004;173:3482–91.

34. Chen Y, Thai P, Zhao YH, et al. Stimulation of airway mucin gene expression by interleukin (IL)-17 through IL-6 paracrine/autocrine loop. J Biol Chem. 2003;278:17036–43.

35. Liang SC, Tan XY, Luxenberg DP, et al. Interleukin (IL)-22 and IL-17 are coexpressed by Th17 cells and cooperatively enhance expression of antimicrobial peptides. J Exp Med. 2006;203:2271–9.

36. Gaffen SL. An overview of IL-17 function and signaling. Cytokine. 2008;43:402–7.

37. Trajkovic V, Stosic-Grujicic S, Samardzic T, et al. Interleukin-17 stimulates inducible nitric oxide synthase activation in rodent astrocytes. J Neuroimmunol. 2001;119:183–91.

38. LeGrand A, Fermor B, Fink C, et al. Interleukin-1, tumor necrosis factor alpha, and interleukin-17 synergistically up-regulate nitric oxide and prostaglandin E2 production in explants of human osteoarthritic knee menisci. Arthritis Rheum. 2001;44:2078–83.

39. Zheng Y, Danilenko DM, Valdez P, et al. Interleukin-22, a T(H)17 cytokine, mediates IL-23-induced dermal inflammation and acanthosis. Nature. 2007;445:648–51.

40. Ganz T. Defensins and host defense. Science. 1999;286:420–1.

41. Oppenheim JJ, Biragyn A, Kwak LW, Yang D. Roles of antimicrobial peptides such as defensins in innate and adaptive immunity. Ann Rheum Dis. 2003;62(Suppl 2):ii17–21.

42. Flo TH, Smith KD, Sato S, et al. Lipocalin 2 mediates an innate immune response to bacterial infection by sequestrating iron. Nature. 2004;432:917–21.

43. Chan YR, Liu JS, Pociask DA, et al. Lipocalin 2 is required for pulmonary host defense against Klebsiella infection. J Immunol. 2009;182:4947–56.
44. Conti HR, Shen F, Nayyar N, et al. Th17 cells and IL-17 receptor signaling are essential for mucosal host defense against oral candidiasis. J Exp Med. 2009;206:299–311.
45. Cho JS, Pietras EM, Garcia NC, et al. IL-17 is essential for host defense against cutaneous *Staphylococcus aureus* infection in mice. J Clin Invest. 2010;120:1762–73.
46. Conti HR, Peterson AC, Brane L, et al. Oral-resident natural Th17 cells and gammadelta T cells control opportunistic *Candida albicans* infections. J Exp Med. 2014;211:2075–84.
47. Bjorses P, Halonen M, Palvimo JJ, et al. Mutations in the AIRE gene: effects on subcellular location and transactivation function of the autoimmune polyendocrinopathy-candidiasis-ectodermal dystrophy protein. Am J Hum Genet. 2000;66:378–92.
48. Oftedal BE, Hellesen A, Erichsen MM, et al. Dominant mutations in the autoimmune regulator AIRE are associated with common organ-specific autoimmune diseases. Immunity. 2015;42:1185–96.
49. Cetani F, Barbesino G, Borsari S, et al. A novel mutation of the autoimmune regulator gene in an Italian kindred with autoimmune polyendocrinopathy-candidiasis-ectodermal dystrophy, acting in a dominant fashion and strongly cosegregating with hypothyroid autoimmune thyroiditis. J Clin Endocrinol Metab. 2001;86:4747–52.
50. The Human Gene Mutation database. http://www.hgmd.cf.ac.uk. Accessed 9 Sep 2016.
51. Puel A, Cypowyj S, Bustamante J, et al. Casanova, Chronic mucocutaneous candidiasis in humans with inborn errors of interleukin-17 immunity. Science. 2011;332:65–8.
52. Ling Y, Cypowyj S, Aytekin C, et al. Inherited IL-17RC deficiency in patients with chronic mucocutaneous candidiasis. J Exp Med. 2015;212:619–31.
53. Boisson B, Wang C, Pedergnana V, et al. An ACT1 mutation selectively abolishes interleukin-17 responses in humans with chronic mucocutaneous candidiasis. Immunity. 2013;39:676–86.
54. Okada S, Markle JG, Deenick EK, et al. Impairment of immunity to Candida and Mycobacterium in humans with bi-allelic RORC mutations. Science. 2015;349:606–13.
55. de Beaucoudrey L, Puel A, Filipe-Santos O, et al. Casanova, Mutations in STAT3 and IL12RB1 impair the development of human IL-17-producing T cells. J Exp Med. 2008;205:1543–50.

56. Ma CS, Chew GY, Simpson N, et al. Deficiency of Th17 cells in hyper IgE syndrome due to mutations in STAT3. J Exp Med. 2008;205:1551–7.

57. Chandesris MO, Melki I, Natividad A, et al. Autosomal dominant STAT3 deficiency and hyper-IgE syndrome: molecular, cellular, and clinical features from a French national survey. Medicine (Baltimore). 2012;91:e1–19.

58. Wilson RP, Ives ML, Rao G, et al. STAT3 is a critical cell-intrinsic regulator of human unconventional T cell numbers and function. J Exp Med. 2015;212:855–64.

59. Zhang LY, Tian W, Shu L, et al. Clinical features, STAT3 gene mutations and Th17 cell analysis in nine children with hyper-IgE syndrome in mainland China. Scand J Immunol. 2013;78: 258–65.

60. Lee WI, Huang JL, Lin SJ, et al. Clinical, immunological and genetic features in Taiwanese patients with the phenotype of hyper-immunoglobulin E recurrent infection syndromes (HIES). Immunobiology. 2011;216:909–17.

61. Milner JD, Brenchley JM, Laurence A, et al. Impaired T(H)17 cell differentiation in subjects with autosomal dominant hyper-IgE syndrome. Nature. 2008;452:773–6.

62. Yamazaki Y, Yamada M, Kawai T, et al. Two novel gain-of-function mutations of STAT1 responsible for chronic mucocutaneous candidiasis disease: impaired production of IL-17A and IL-22, and the presence of anti-IL-17F autoantibody. J Immunol. 2014;193:4880–7.

63. Liu L, Okada S, Kong XF, et al. Gain-of-function human STAT1 mutations impair IL-17 immunity and underlie chronic mucocutaneous candidiasis. J Exp Med. 2011;208:1635–48.

64. Martinez-Martinez L, Martinez-Saavedra MT, Fuentes-Prior P, et al. A novel gain-of-function STAT1 mutation resulting in basal phosphorylation of STAT1 and increased distal IFN-gamma-mediated responses in chronic mucocutaneous candidiasis. Mol Immunol. 2015;68:597–605.

65. Drummond RA, Lionakis MS. Mechanistic insights into the role of C-type lectin receptor/CARD9 signaling in human antifungal immunity. Front Cell Infect Microbiol. 2016;6:39.

66. Ferwerda B, Ferwerda G, Plantinga TS, et al. Human dectin-1 deficiency and mucocutaneous fungal infections. N Engl J Med. 2009;361:1760–7.

67. Plantinga TS, van der Velden WJ, Ferwerda B, et al. Early stop polymorphism in human DECTIN-1 is associated with increased

candida colonization in hematopoietic stem cell transplant recipients. Clin Infect Dis. 2009;49:724–32.

68. Kreins AY, Ciancanelli MJ, Okada S, et al. Human TYK2 deficiency: mycobacterial and viral infections without hyper-IgE syndrome. J Exp Med. 2015;212:1641–62.

69. Prando C, Samarina A, Bustamante J, et al. Inherited IL-12p40 deficiency: genetic, immunologic, and clinical features of 49 patients from 30 kindreds. Medicine (Baltimore). 2013;92:109–22.

70. de Beaucoudrey L, Samarina A, Bustamante J, et al. Revisiting human IL-12Rbeta1 deficiency: a survey of 141 patients from 30 countries. Medicine (Baltimore). 2010;89:381–402.

71. Ouederni M, Sanal O, Ikinciogullari A, et al. Clinical features of Candidiasis in patients with inherited interleukin 12 receptor beta1 deficiency. Clin Infect Dis. 2014;58:204–13.

72. Patel DD, Kuchroo VK. Th17 cell pathway in human immunity: Lessons from Genetics and Therapeutic Interventions. Immunity. 2015;43:1040–51.

73. Whibley N, Tritto E, Traggiai E, et al. Antibody blockade of IL-17 family cytokines in immunity to acute murine oral mucosal candidiasis. J Leukoc Biol. 2016;99:1153–64.

74. Huang W, Na L, Fidel PL, Schwarzenberger P. Requirement of interleukin-17 A for systemic anti-*Candida albicans* host defense in mice. J Infect Dis. 2004;190:624–31.

75. Bar E, Whitney PG, Moor K, Reis e Sousa C, LeibundGut-Landmann S. IL-17 regulates systemic fungal immunity by controlling the functional competence of NK cells. Immunity. 2014;40:117–27.

Chapter 3
Th17 Cells: Differentiation and Regulation

3.1 Identification of Th17 Cells

The increased IL-17A production by CD4+ T cells from T cell receptor (TCR) transgenic DO11.10 mice was first observed by Infante-Duarte and colleagues in 2000 [1]. The transgenic TCR recognizes ovalbumin (OVA) peptide 322-339 in association with I-A^d. When stimulated with OVA$_{322-339}$ in the presence of cell lysates of *Borrelia burgdorferi*, these CD4+ Th cells preferentially produce IL-17A along with tumor necrosis factor (TNF) and granulocyte-macrophage colony-stimulating factor (GM-CSF). The cytokine profile produced by these CD4+ Th cells is distinctive from those by Th1 or Th2 cells. Interleukin 6 (IL-6) was shown to have a similar effect to cell lysates of *Borrelia burgdorferi* in inducing IL-17A production by these CD4+ Th cells. In 2003, Aggarwal et al. [2] showed that IL-23 preferentially promotes IL-17A and IL-17F production by activated CD4+ T cells in vitro suggesting that during a secondary immune response IL-23 can promote a distinct differentiation status from well-characterized Th1 and Th2 cells. In an experimental autoimmune encephalomyelitis (EAE) model, Cua and colleagues demonstrated that it is IL-23 rather than IL-12 mediating autoimmune inflammation of the brain [3]. Furthermore, they provided in vivo evidence that IL-23 drives a pathogenic T cell population mediating inflammation in EAE and arthritis models [2, 4]. These

C.-Q. Chu, *Targeting the IL-17 Pathway in Inflammatory Disorders*, DOI 10.1007/978-3-319-28040-0_3,
© Springer International Publishing Switzerland 2017

pathogenic CD4$^+$ T cells produce IL-17A, IL-17F, IL-6, and TNF. The term "Th17 cells" was proposed in 2005 by two independent groups led by Dong and Weaver, respectively [5, 6], to describe a Th cell lineage, which is distinctive from Th1 and Th2 cells. A Th17 cell is governed by its master transcription factor, retinoic acid receptor-related orphan nuclear receptor (ROR)-γt [7]. The discovery of Th17 cells heralded a major shift in T cell biology and our understanding of the mechanism of autoimmune inflammatory diseases. Cytokines produced by Th17 cells include IL-17A, IL-17F, IL-22, GM-CSF, IL-21, and TNF depending on inflammatory settings [8]. Those autoimmune diseases thought to be mediated by Th1 cells are now recognized to be mediated mainly by Th17 cells [9].

3.2   Cytokines Promoting Th17 Cell Differentiation

It has been clearly demonstrated by in vitro experiments that several cytokines are involved in promoting differentiation and development of Th17 cells. These include IL-6, IL-1, TNF, GM-CSF, transforming growth factor (TGF)-β, and IL-23. IL-6 is one of the cytokines involved in the initiation of CD4$^+$ T cell differentiation toward Th17 cells (see Fig. 3.1) [10–12] in the presence of TGF-β.

As described above, IL-6 can replace lysates of *Borrelia burgdorferi* to promote OVA$_{322\text{-}339}$-specific CD4$^+$ Th cells to produce IL-17A [1]. This suggests that IL-6 drives activation of a unique pathway leading to expression of IL-17A by CD4$^+$ Th cells. Subsequent experiments indicate that IL-6 is essential in this process by activating signal transducers and activators of transcription (STAT)-3, which directly activates RORγt [13]. STAT-3 also suppresses TGF-β-induced forkhead box P3 (FOXP3) expression and thereby inhibits the CD4$^+$ Th differentiation toward T regulatory (Treg) cell lineage [13, 14]. IL-6 also promotes IL-23 receptor expression by these CD4$^+$ T cells (Fig. 3.1) and thereby potentiates these Th17 cells to receive signals from IL-23 [14, 16]. The essential

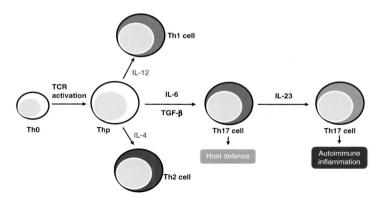

FIGURE 3.1 Development of Th17 cells. Schematic diagram simplified the in vitro model of Th17 cell differentiation and development. A naive CD4+ T cell (Th0) is activated upon T cell antigen receptor (TCR) stimulation and becomes a T helper cell precursor (Thp). A Thp cell can differentiate into different subsets of Th cell depending on different cytokines it encounters. In the presence of TGF-β and IL-6, the Thp cell can differentiate into a Th17 cell that may be important for host defense but may become pathogenic if it is further stimulated by IL-23

role of IL-6 in generating Th17 cells is confirmed in vivo. Activation of STAT3 by inflammatory stimulus is impaired in IL-6 gene knockout mice, fails to develop Th17 cells, and is protected from development of EAE [16] and collagen-induced arthritis (CIA) [17, 18].

IL-1β also has a crucial role in the initiation of Th17 cell differentiation. IL-1R1 knockout mice fail to develop antigen-specific Th17 cells and do not develop EAE [19]. IL-1R1 expression on Th17 cells is induced by IL-6. IL-1 signaling promotes the transcription factor interferon-regulatory factor 4 (IRF4), which further reinforces the expression of RORγt [20]. Mammalian target of rapamycin (mTOR) is essential for IL-1β-induced Th17 proliferation. Thus, mTOR-deficient Th17 cells fail to proliferate in response to IL-1β. IL-1β induces phosphorylation of mTOR [21]. These results suggest that IL-6 directs the initial differentiation of

Th17 cells, while IL-1β promotes the expansion of these cells when they are in competition with other T cell subsets in the context of a resource-limited tissue environment [22].

Involvement of GM-CSF in driving Th17 cells was first demonstrated in an experimental autoimmune myocarditis (EAM) model [23]. Development of EAM is a Th17 cell-mediated disease [24] and is IL-6- and IL-23-dependent [25, 26]. Mice deficient in GM-CSF fail to generate Th17 cells and do not develop EAM. This is the result of diminished production of IL-6 and IL-23 by dendritic cells [23]. Interestingly, GM-CSF deficiency did not affect the development of Th1 or Th2 cells. These results indicate that GM-CSF promotes Th17 cells by indirectly inducing IL-6 and IL-23 production by dendritic cells. GM-CSF is also an important Th17 cell effector cytokine, which is required to mediate inflammation in the EAE model. Recently, it was found that synovial CD4+ Th17 cells in patients with rheumatoid arthritis (RA) produce GM-CSF, which is able to induce an inflammatory dendritic cell phenotype from monocytes [27]. These results suggest a GM-CSF-driven positive feedback loop in operation in RA joints to perpetuate pathogenic Th17 cells.

IL-21 is produced by natural killer (NK) cells and T cells. IL-21 signals through a unique IL-21R chain and the shared common γ-chain (shared by IL-2, IL-4, IL-7, IL-9, and IL-15). IL-21 is an autocrine growth cytokine for the expansion of Th17 cells. IL-21 together with TGF-α is able to induce the differentiation of Th17 cells, and IL-21 can replace IL-6 in this process [28]. In the absence of IL-6, IL-21 together with TGF-α was able to inhibit the development of inducible Treg and to promote the differentiation of Th17 cells [28]. During the initial Th17 differentiation, IL-6-induced IL-21 acts as a positive amplification loop to enforce Th17 differentiation [29, 30]. In vivo, however, the role of IL-21 in the induction of Th17 cells remains controversial. It was reported that the absence of IL-21 or IL-21R had no significant difference on the development of Th17 cells [31, 32]. Thus, IL-21 might be an alternative pathway in inducing and expanding Th17 cells [33].

TGF-β is generally considered an anti-inflammatory cytokine. The role of TGF-β in Th17 cell differentiation is

complex. The effect of TGF-β on promoting IL-17A production by CD4+ T cells was first described by Veldhoen et al.
[12]. TGF-β in combination with IL-6 initiates naive CD4+ T
cells to differentiate into IL-17A-producing cells. This effect
is amplified by IL-1β and TNF [12]. T cell-specific deletion of
the TGF-β gene and expression of the nonfunctional TGF-β
receptor confirmed that endogenous TGF-β induces Th17 cell
development in vivo [34–36]. One caveat associated with
deficient TGF-β signaling is excessive production of IL-4 and
interferon (IFN)-γ, which are potent suppressors of Th17 cell
development and population expansion [34, 35]. So the alternative explanation is that TGF-β indirectly induces Th17
development by suppressing Th1 or Th2 development. Indeed,
in some experiments, in the absence TGF-β, when IL-4 and
IFN-γ activities are neutralized, Th17 cell differentiation can
be initiated and fully developed when IL-23 is added [5, 6].
These results suggest that TGF-β can be spared in the initiation of Th17 differentiation. That is, IL-6 alone can induce
Th17 cell development in T-bet- and STAT6-deficient mice
[37]. In humans, conflicting results were generated in studies
of in vitro development of Th17 cells from naive CD4+ T cells
by different groups. Thus, TGF-β is dispensable to development of Th17 cells in some but not in the other experiments
[38–42]. Interestingly, Th17 cells generated by TGF-β and
IL-6 are less pathogenic. In contrast, Th17 cells generated by
IL-6 and IL-23 are highly pathogenic and able to induce
severe EAE [15].

The role of IL-23 in Th17 cell survival is indispensable [2, 4].
Mice with the IL-23 p19 gene knockout generate no or few
Th17 cells and do not develop EAE or CIA [2, 4]. However,
IL-23 is not required for the initial differentiation of Th17 cells,
but is essential for clonal expansion and stabilization of Th17
cells [12]. Naive CD4+ T cells do not express IL-23R. IL-23
alone cannot initiate the differentiation of Th17 cells from
naive CD4+ T cell precursors [2, 10]. Earlier studies indicate
that IL-23 acts on activated and memory CD4+ T cells to
induce IL-17A production [1]. Upon IL-6-mediated initial differentiation, Th17 cells express IL-23R [15]. IL-23 signaling
further increases IL-23R expression (Fig. 3.1) [15] to reinforce

the action of IL-23 on Th17 cells. This fact is particularly relevant to therapeutic strategy design for targeting IL-17/Th17 pathway. In Th17 cell-mediated disease, pathogenic Th17 cells are already formed and need constant IL-23 signaling for survival. Therefore, interrupted IL-23 signaling would be effective to eliminate pathogenic Th17 cells. It has been suggested that Th17 cells activated by TGF-β and IL-6 play a more physiological role in mucosal defense and barrier tissue integrity and may also curtail immunopathogenic responses (Fig. 3.1) [43–45], while IL-23-activated Th17 cells play a role in chronic tissue inflammation during infection, granuloma formation, and autoimmune conditions (Fig. 3.1). These have been demonstrated in experiments in neutralizing IL-23 activity in disease models [46, 47] and provide evidence for the rationale of IL-23-targeted therapy in human disease (see below).

In summary, data from in vitro and in vivo experiments indicate that TGF-β, IL-6, and IL-1β are essential cytokines that initiate Th17 cell differentiation; IL-21 drives Th17 cell growth in an autocrine fashion; GM-CSF is a Th17 effector cytokine, which also promotes Th17 cell differentiation; and IL-23 is the cytokine that promotes Th17 cell differentiation and is essential for the pathogenic inflammatory function of Th17 cells.

3.3   Cytokines Suppressing Th17 Cells

IL-27 is a heterodimeric cytokine comprised of Epstein–Barr virus-induced gene 3 (*EBI3*) and IL-27p28 subunits. IL-27 signals through IL-27Rα and gp130 [48]. IL-27 is a potent inhibitor of IL-17 production. IL-27 receptor-deficient mice infected with *Toxoplasma gondii* develop severe neuroinflammation, which is mediated by Th17 cells [49]. In vitro, IL-27 is able to completely suppress IL-6 and TGF-β–induced de novo Th17 differentiation but has a lesser inhibitory effect to counter IL-23-mediated development of Th17 cells [49–51]. IL-27 fails to suppress IL-17A from encephalitogenic Th17 cells [50]. These results suggest that IL-27 may have an impact during Th17 differentiation but have a limited effect on already committed Th17 cells.

The role of IFN-γ in Th17 cells is complex. Historically, IFN-γ was considered the effector cytokine of Th1 cells mediating many of the autoimmune inflammatory diseases, which are now confirmed to be mediated by Th17 cells. IFN-γ knockout mice develop severe EAE and CIA with increased number of Th17 cells [52–54]. Arthritis in IFN-γ-deficient mice is suppressed by neutralizing IL-17A antibodies [53]. In vitro de novo differentiation of Th17 cells is suppressed by the presence of IFN-γ [5, 6]. These results clearly indicate the inhibitory effect of IFN-γ on the development of Th17 cells. However, other studies provided evidence indicating that IFN-γ might be required for pathogenicity of Th17 cells [15, 55, 56]. Those Th17 cells inducing EAE co-express IFN-γ. IL-17A and IFN-γ co-expressing Th17 cells also exist in human diseases [57, 58]. It appears that the so-called Th17 cells are plastic and are able to shift toward Th1-like cells [24, 45, 59–61]. In humans, those IL-17A and IFN-γ co-expressing Th17 cells may represent a transient status of the Th17 cells and are dependent on DNA methylation status of *Rorc2* and *Il17a* genes [62]. The heterogeneity of Th17 cells may originate from the Th17 precursors, which are CD4$^+$ CD161$^+$. These CD4$^+$ CD161$^+$-naive T cells can be differentiated into Th17 cells or non-classic Th1 cells, which express RORγt but are able to produce IFN-γ as well as IL-17A [62, 63]. However, whether and how much IFN-γ contributes to the pathogenicity of these Th17 cells is unclear and is difficult to delineate with certainty.

The signature Th2 cytokine, IL-4, is also a potent inhibitor of Th17 cells [5, 6]. IL-4-mediated inhibition of Th17 cells is STAT6 dependent but not GATA3 dependent. The inhibitory effect of IL-4 takes effect during the initial de novo differentiation stage but has no impact on fully differentiated Th17 cells [64]. This highlights that as with IL-27, IL-4 may only have limited application as a therapeutic agent to treat Th17-mediated conditions.

3.4   Transcriptional Regulation of Th17 Cells

The differentiation and development Th17 cells are finely controlled by transcription factors (Fig. 3.2).

Of these transcription factors, RORγt is the master controller to determine the CD4⁺ T cell fate to become Th17 cells. ROR are members of the nuclear receptor family of intracellular transcription factors [65, 66]. The ROR subfamily has three members in mammals: RORα, RORβ, and RORγ [67]. RORγ is encoded by the *Rorc* gene. RORγ is expressed in many tissues such as the heart, kidney, liver, lung, brain, and muscle. RORγt was first identified by He et al. [68] as a thymus-specific isoform of RORγ that is expressed predominantly in CD4⁺ CD8⁺ double-positive

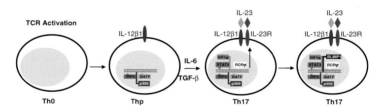

FIGURE 3.2 Transcriptional regulation of Th17 cells. Many transcription factors are involved in the regulation of Th17 cell differentiation and development. IRF4 and BATF bind *Il17a* promoter upon TCR activation and allow other lineage-specific transcription factors to access the chromatin. STAT3 is recruited by IL-6 to promote Rorc expression. HIF1α and RORγt form a complex to drive IL-17A expression. RORγt directly controls *Il17a*, *Il17f*, and *Il23r* genes but not other genes. This renders RORγt an excellent drug target for suppressing Th17 cells without affecting other cell types. *BATF* basic leucine zipper transcription factor, ATF-like, *BLIMP1* B lymphocyte-induced maturation protein 1 (also known as PRDM1, PR domain zinc finger protein 1), *HIF1α* hypoxia-inducible factor 1α, *IRF4* interferon regulatory factor 4, *RORγt* retinoic acid receptor (RAR)-related orphan receptor-γt, *STAT* signal transducers and activators of transcription, *TCR* T cell antigen receptor, *Thp* T helper cell precursor

thymocytes [69]. In fact, RORγt is a splice variant of RORγ, which is different only at the N-terminus [68]. Unlike the wide tissue expression of RORγ, RORγt is expressed exclusively in lymphoid cells [70]. RORγt is critical in regulating gene expression during the development of T cells and the formation of the secondary lymphoid organ [71–73]. *Rorc* gene-deficient CD4+CD8+ thymocytes undergo early apoptosis, and the animals fail to develop lymph nodes, Peyer's patches, and lymphoid tissue inducer cells (LTi) [72, 73]. In vitro, as a result of the absence of *Rorc* in CD4+ T cells, IL-17 expression was greatly impaired under Th17-polarizing conditions. This has been seen in humans with RORγt deficiency [74]. Conversely, overexpression of RORγt in naive CD4+ T cells was sufficient to induce the expression of IL-17A, IL-17F, and IL-22 [7]. RORγt is essential for the expression of IL-17 as well as the differentiation of Th17 in mouse and human CD4+ T cells [7, 39]. RORγ-deficient mice produce few Th17 cells and fail to develop EAE [7]. Therefore, the role of RORγt is similar to transcription factors such as T-bet and GATA3 in Th1 and Th2 differentiation, respectively, and hence, RORγt is the master transcriptional factor for Th17 differentiation [60, 75]. Agents targeting RORγt are effective in inhibiting Th17 differentiation and suppression of disease models of inflammation (see below). RORγt promotes IL-17 expression by directly binding the promotor region of *Il17* genes at multiple sites [7, 76, 77].

Another related retinoic acid nuclear receptor, RORα, is also expressed in Th17 cells both in vitro and in vivo. RORα expression is induced by TGF-β and IL-6 via STAT3. CD4+ T cells deficient in *Rora* have impaired Th17 differentiation but are not completely abolished. Mice deficient in RORα produce fewer Th17 cells in vivo and develop less severe EAE, but disease incidence was not affected [78]. Interestingly, RORα deficiency impairs IL-17A but not IL-17F expression. Co-overexpression of RORα and RORγ significantly increases Th17 differentiation [79]. These results suggest that RORα is a transcription factor that synergizes RORγt function but is not essential for Th17 cell differentiation.

The transcription factor STAT3, which is preferentially activated by IL-6, IL-21, and IL-23, is capable of inducing RORγt and regulating Th17 cell development [13, 80]. Deficiency of STAT3 in CD4+ T cells impaired Th17 cell differentiation in vivo, and overexpression of a constitutively active STAT3 could increase IL-17A production [13, 81]. STAT3 might affect the production of IL-17 by increasing the expression of RORγt and RORα [13, 78]. Furthermore, STAT3 also binds directly to the *Il17* and *Il21* promoters and leads to the expression of IL-17A and IL-21 [82, 83]. Therefore, STAT3 and RORγt seem to cooperate to induce IL-17A production.

Earlier studies have demonstrated that multiple other transcription factors also participate in regulating the development of Th17 cells. These include IRF4, BATF, and RUNX1 [75]. The importance of IRF4 and BATF was confirmed by a gene-deficient approach. BATF-deficient CD4+ T cells fail to maintain RORγt expression, and mice with BATF deficiency are resistant to induction of EAE [84]. Similarly, IRF4-deficient mice were shown to have impaired Th17 responses and were resistant to EAE [85]. Interestingly, deficiency in either of BATF or IRF4 results in defective Th1, Th2, Th9, and T follicular helper (Tfh) cell development [86–89]. Several studies indicate that in the early event of Th0 activation, BATF and IRF4 cooperate to allow the accessibility of chromatin by other lineage-specific transcription factors to determine the fate of Th cell differentiation. During Th17 cell differentiation, upon TCR signaling, the so-called pioneer factors, BATF and IRF4, bind *Il17a* gene promoter region and regulatory enhancer in multiple sites [90, 91]. IL-6 signaling recruits STAT3, BATF, IRF4, and STAT3 complex along the co-activator histone acetyltransferase p300 to promote the expression of *Rorc* [91]. TCR and IL-6 signaling also promotes the expression if hypoxia-inducible factor 1α (HIF1α), a key sensor of hypoxia [92]. HIF1α directly binds and drives transcription of *Rorc* and forms a complex with RORγt and p300 to drive *Il17* gene expression. HIF1α also binds to FOXP3 to induce proteasomal degradation of FOXP3 [92].

IRF4, BATF, STAT3, RORγt, and HIF1α complex further induces expression of *Il23r*. This allows IL-23 to induce maturation of Th17 cells. IL-23 signaling activates and recruits B lymphocyte-induced maturation protein 1 (BLIMP1) to the STAT3-RORγt transcription factor complex to enhance the expression of Th17 cell signature genes (Fig. 3.2) [22].

It is interesting to note that RORγt only directly controls *Il17a*, *Il17f*, and *Il23r* genes. For example, a lack of RORγt does not affect p300 recruitment. This renders RORγt an exceptional drug target as therapeutic intervention would not be expected to perturb the genetic regulatory programs shared by other cell types [91].

References

1. Gaffen SL. An overview of IL-17 function and signaling. Cytokine. 2008;43:402–7.
2. Aggarwal S, Ghilardi N, Xie MH, de Sauvage FJ, Gurney AL. Interleukin-23 promotes a distinct CD4 T cell activation state characterized by the production of interleukin-17. J Biol Chem. 2003;278(3):1910–4.
3. Infante-Duarte C, Horton HF, Byrne MC, Kamradt T. Microbial lipopeptides induce the production of IL-17 in Th cells. J Immunol. 2000;165:6107–15.
4. Cua DJ, Sherlock J, Chen Y, Murphy CA, Joyce B, Seymour B, Lucian L, W. To, Kwan S, Churakova T, Zurawski S, Wiekowski M, Lira SA, Gorman D, Kastelein RA, Sedgwick JD. Interleukin-23 rather than interleukin-12 is the critical cytokine for autoimmune inflammation of the brain. Nature. 2003;421:744–8.
5. Langrish CL, Chen Y, Blumenschein WM, et al. IL-23 drives a pathogenic T cell population that induces autoimmune inflammation. J Exp Med. 2005;201:233–40.
6. Murphy CA, Langrish CL, Chen Y, et al. Divergent pro- and anti-inflammatory roles for IL-23 and IL-12 in joint autoimmune inflammation. J Exp Med. 2003;198:1951–7.
7. Harrington LE, Hatton RD, Mangan PR, et al. Interleukin 17-producing CD4+ effector T cells develop via a lineage distinct from the T helper type 1 and 2 lineages. Nat Immunol. 2005;6: 1123–32.

8. Hirota K, Ahlfors H, Duarte JH, Stockinger B. Regulation and function of innate and adaptive interleukin-17-producing cells. EMBO Rep. 2012;13:113–20.
9. Park H, Li Z, Yang XO, et al. A distinct lineage of CD4 T cells regulates tissue inflammation by producing interleukin 17. Nat Immunol. 2005;6:1133–41.
10. Ivanov II, McKenzie BS, Zhou L, et al. The orphan nuclear receptor RORgammat directs the differentiation program of proinflammatory IL-17+ T helper cells. Cell. 2006;126:1121–33.
11. Watford WT, O'Shea JJ. Autoimmunity: a case of mistaken identity. Nature. 2003;421:706–8.
12. Bettelli E, Carrier Y, Gao W, et al. Reciprocal developmental pathways for the generation of pathogenic effector TH17 and regulatory T cells. Nature. 2006;441:235–8.
13. Mangan PR, Harrington LE, O'Quinn DB, et al. Transforming growth factor-beta induces development of the T(H)17 lineage. Nature. 2006;441:231–4.
14. Veldhoen M, Hocking RJ, Atkins CJ, Locksley RM, Stockinger B. TGFbeta in the context of an inflammatory cytokine milieu supports de novo differentiation of IL-17-producing T cells. Immunity. 2006;24:179–89.
15. Yang XO, Panopoulos AD, Nurieva R, et al. STAT3 regulates cytokine-mediated generation of inflammatory helper T cells. J Biol Chem. 2007;282:9358–63.
16. Durant L, Watford WT, Ramos HL, et al. Diverse targets of the transcription factor STAT3 contribute to T cell pathogenicity and homeostasis. Immunity. 2010;32:605–15.
17. Ghoreschi K, Laurence A, Yang XP, et al. Generation of pathogenic T(H)17 cells in the absence of TGF-beta signaling. Nature. 2010;467:967–71.
18. Samoilova EB, Horton JL, Hilliard B, Liu TS, Chen Y. IL-6-deficient mice are resistant to experimental autoimmune encephalomyelitis: roles of IL-6 in the activation and differentiation of autoreactive T cells. J Immunol. 1998;161:6480–6.
19. Alonzi T, Fattori E, Lazzaro D, et al. Interleukin 6 is required for the development of collagen-induced arthritis. J Exp Med. 1998;187:461–8.
20. Alonzi T, Fattori E, Cappelletti M, Ciliberto G, Poli V. Impaired Stat3 activation following localized inflammatory stimulus in IL-6-deficient mice. Cytokine. 1998;10:13–8.
21. Sutton C, Brereton C, Keogh B, Mills KH, Lavelle EC. A crucial role for interleukin (IL)-1 in the induction of IL-17-producing T

cells that mediate autoimmune encephalomyelitis. J Exp Med. 2006;203:1685–91.

22. Chung Y, Chang SH, Martinez GJ, et al. Critical regulation of early Th17 cell differentiation by interleukin-1 signaling. Immunity. 2009;30:576–87.

23. Gulen MF, Kang Z, Bulek K, et al. The receptor SIGIRR suppresses Th17 cell proliferation via inhibition of the interleukin-1 receptor pathway and mTOR kinase activation. Immunity. 2010;32:54–66.

24. Gaffen SL, Jain R, Garg AV, Cua DJ. The IL-23-IL-17 immune axis: from mechanisms to therapeutic testing. Nat Rev Immunol. 2014;14:585–600.

25. Sonderegger I, Iezzi G, Maier R, Schmitz N, Kurrer M, Kopf M. GM-CSF mediates autoimmunity by enhancing IL-6-dependent Th17 cell development and survival. J Exp Med. 2008;205: 2281–94.

26. Yamashita T, Iwakura T, Matsui K, et al. IL-6-mediated Th17 differentiation through RORgammat is essential for the initiation of experimental autoimmune myocarditis. Cardiovasc Res. 2011;91:640–8.

27. Sonderegger I, Rohn TA, Kurrer MO, et al. Neutralization of IL-17 by active vaccination inhibits IL-23-dependent autoimmune myocarditis. Eur J Immunol. 2006;36:2849–56.

28. Eriksson U, Kurrer MO, Schmitz N, et al. Interleukin-6-deficient mice resist development of autoimmune myocarditis associated with impaired upregulation of complement C3. Circulation. 2003;107:320–5.

29. Reynolds G, Gibbon JR, Pratt AG, et al. Synovial CD4+ T-cell-derived GM-CSF supports the differentiation of an inflammatory dendritic cell population in rheumatoid arthritis. Ann Rheum Dis. 2016;75:899–907.

30. Korn T, Bettelli E, Gao W, et al. IL-21 initiates an alternative pathway to induce proinflammatory T(H)17 cells. Nature. 2007;448:484–7.

31. Nurieva R, Yang XO, Martinez G, et al. Essential autocrine regulation by IL-21 in the generation of inflammatory T cells. Nature. 2007;448:480–3.

32. Zhou L, Ivanov II, Spolski R, et al. IL-6 programs T(H)-17 cell differentiation by promoting sequential engagement of the IL-21 and IL-23 pathways. Nat Immunol. 2007;8:967–74.

33. Coquet JM, Chakravarti S, Smyth MJ, Godfrey DI. Cutting edge: IL-21 is not essential for Th17 differentiation or experimental autoimmune encephalomyelitis. J Immunol. 2008;180:7097–101.

34. Liu R, Bai Y, Vollmer TL, et al. IL-21 receptor expression deter-mines the temporal phases of experimental autoimmune enceph-alomyelitis. Exp Neurol. 2008;211:14–24.
35. Korn T, Bettelli E, Oukka M, Kuchroo VK. IL-17 and Th17 cells. Annu Rev Immunol. 2009;27:485–517.
36. Veldhoen M, Hocking RJ, Flavell RA, Stockinger B. Signals mediated by transforming growth factor-beta initiate autoimmune encephalomyelitis, but chronic inflammation is needed to sustain disease. Nat Immunol. 2006;7:1151–6.
37. Li MO, Wan YY, Flavell RA. T cell-produced transforming growth factor-beta1 controls T cell tolerance and regulates Th1- and Th17-cell differentiation. Immunity. 2007;26:579–91.
38. Gutcher I, Donkor MK, Ma Q, Rudensky AY, Flavell RA, Li MO. Autocrine transforming growth factor-beta1 promotes in vivo Th17 cell differentiation. Immunity. 2011;34:396–408.
39. Das J, Ren G, Zhang L, Roberts AI, et al. Transforming growth factor beta is dispensable for the molecular orchestration of Th17 cell differentiation. J Exp Med. 2009;206:2407–16.
40. Volpe E, Servant N, Zollinger R, et al. A critical function for transforming growth factor-beta, interleukin 23 and proinflam-matory cytokines in driving and modulating human T(H)-17 responses. Nat Immunol. 2008;9:650–7.
41. Manel N, Unutmaz D, Littman DR. The differentiation of human T(H)-17 cells requires transforming growth factor-beta and induction of the nuclear receptor RORgammat. Nat Immunol. 2008;9:641–9.
42. Acosta-Rodriguez EV, Napolitani G, Lanzavecchia A, Sallusto F. Interleukins 1beta and 6 but not transforming growth factor-beta are essential for the differentiation of interleukin 17-producing human T helper cells. Nat Immunol. 2007;8:942–9.
43. Wilson NJ, Boniface K, Chan JR, et al. Development, cytokine profile and function of human interleukin 17-producing helper T cells. Nat Immunol. 2007;8:950–7.
44. Chen Z, Tato CM, Muul L, Laurence A, O'Shea JJ. Distinct regu-lation of interleukin-17 in human T helper lymphocytes. Arthritis Rheum. 2007;56:2936–46.
45. McGeachy MJ, Bak-Jensen KS, Chen Y, Tato CM, et al. TGF-beta and IL-6 drive the production of IL-17 and IL-10 by T cells and restrain T(H)-17 cell-mediated pathology. Nat Immunol. 2007;8:1390–7.

46. Hirota K, Turner JE, Villa M, et al. Plasticity of Th17 cells in Peyer's patches is responsible for the induction of T cell-dependent IgA responses. Nat Immunol. 2013;14:372–9.

47. Esplugues E, Huber S, Gagliani N, et al. Control of TH17 cells occurs in the small intestine. Nature. 2011;475:514–8.

48. Chackerian AA, Chen SJ, Brodie SJ, et al. Neutralization or absence of the interleukin-23 pathway does not compromise immunity to mycobacterial infection. Infect Immun. 2006;74:6092–9.

49. Chen Y, Langrish CL, McKenzie B, et al. Anti-IL-23 therapy inhibits multiple inflammatory pathways and ameliorates autoimmune encephalomyelitis. J Clin Invest. 2006;116:1317–26.

50. Yoshida H, Hunter CA. The immunobiology of interleukin-27. Annu Rev Immunol. 2015;33:417–43.

51. Stumhofer JS, Laurence A, Wilson EH, et al. Interleukin 27 negatively regulates the development of interleukin 17-producing T helper cells during chronic inflammation of the central nervous system. Nat Immunol. 2006;7:937–45.

52. El-behi M, Ciric B, Yu S, et al. Differential effect of IL-27 on developing versus committed Th17 cells. J Immunol. 2009; 183:4957–67.

53. Hirahara K, Ghoreschi K, Yang XP, et al. Interleukin-27 priming of T cells controls IL-17 production in trans via induction of the ligand PD-L1. Immunity. 2012;36:1017–30.

54. Chu CQ, Song Z, Mayton L, Wu B, Wooley PH. IFNgamma deficient C57BL/6 (H-2b) mice develop collagen induced arthritis with predominant usage of T cell receptor Vbeta6 and Vbeta8 in arthritic joints. Ann Rheum Dis. 2003;62:983–90.

55. Chu CQ, Swart D, Alcorn D, Tocker J, Elkon KB. Interferon-gamma regulates susceptibility to collagen-induced arthritis through suppression of interleukin-17. Arthritis Rheum. 2007;56: 1145–51.

56. Chu CQ, Wittmer S, Dalton DK. Failure to suppress the expansion of the activated CD4 T cell population in interferon gamma-deficient mice leads to exacerbation of experimental autoimmune encephalomyelitis. J Exp Med. 2000;192:123–8.

57. Haines CJ, Chen Y, Blumenschein WM, et al. Autoimmune memory T helper 17 cell function and expansion are dependent on interleukin-23. Cell Rep. 2013;3:1378–88.

58. Haines CJ, Cua DJ. Orphan cytokine reveals IL-17 family secret. Immunity. 2011;35:498–500.

59. Kebir H, Ifergan I, Alvarez JI, et al. Preferential recruitment of interferon-gamma-expressing TH17 cells in multiple sclerosis. Ann Neurol. 2009;66:390–402.
60. Nistala K, Adams S, Cambrook H, et al. Th17 plasticity in human autoimmune arthritis is driven by the inflammatory environment. Proc Natl Acad Sci U S A. 2010;107:14751–6.
61. Hirota K, Duarte JH, Veldhoen M, et al. Fate mapping of IL-17-producing T cells in inflammatory responses. Nat Immunol. 2011;12:255–63.
62. Lee Y, Awasthi A, Yosef N, et al. Induction and molecular signature of pathogenic TH17 cells. Nat Immunol. 2012;13:991–9.
63. Yang XO, Nurieva R, Martinez GJ, et al. Molecular antagonism and plasticity of regulatory and inflammatory T cell programs. Immunity. 2008;29:44–56.
64. Mazzoni A, Santarlasci V, Maggi L, et al. Demethylation of the RORC2 and IL17A in human CD4+ T lymphocytes defines Th17 origin of nonclassic Th1 cells. J Immunol. 2015;194:3116–26.
65. Cosmi L, De Palma R, Santarlasci V, et al. Human interleukin 17-producing cells originate from a CD161+CD4+ T cell precursor. J Exp Med. 2008;205:1903–16.
66. Cooney LA, Towery K, Endres J, Fox DA. Sensitivity and resistance to regulation by IL-4 during Th17 maturation. J Immunol. 2011;187:4440–50.
67. Giguere V. Retinoic acid receptors and cellular retinoid binding proteins: complex interplay in retinoid signaling. Endocr Rev. 1994;15:61–79.
68. Hirose T, Smith RJ, Jetten AM. ROR gamma: the third member of ROR/RZR orphan receptor subfamily that is highly expressed in skeletal muscle. Biochem Biophys Res Commun. 1994;205:1976–83.
69. Jetten AM. Retinoid-related orphan receptors (RORs): critical roles in development, immunity, circadian rhythm, and cellular metabolism. Nucl Recept Signal. 2009;7:e003.
70. He YW, Deftos ML, Ojala EW, Bevan MJ. RORgamma t, a novel isoform of an orphan receptor, negatively regulates Fas ligand expression and IL-2 production in T cells. Immunity. 1998;9:797–806.
71. He YW, Beers C, Deftos ML, Ojala EW, Forbush KA, Bevan MJ. Down-regulation of the orphan nuclear receptor ROR gamma t is essential for T lymphocyte maturation. J Immunol. 2000;164:5668–74.

72. Eberl G, Littman DR. The role of the nuclear hormone receptor RORgammat in the development of lymph nodes and Peyer's patches. Immunol Rev. 2003;195:81–90.

73. Eberl G, Marmon S, Sunshine MJ, Rennert PD, Choi Y, Littman DR. An essential function for the nuclear receptor RORgamma(t) in the generation of fetal lymphoid tissue inducer cells. Nat Immunol. 2004;5:64–73.

74. Okada S, Markle JG, Deenick EK, et al. Impairment of immunity to Candida and Mycobacterium in humans with bi-allelic RORC mutations. Science. 2015;349:606–13.

75. Kurebayashi S, Ueda E, Sakaue M, et al. Retinoid-related orphan receptor gamma (RORgamma) is essential for lymphoid organogenesis and controls apoptosis during thymopoiesis. Proc Natl Acad Sci U S A. 2000;97:10132–7.

76. Sun Z, Unutmaz D, Zou YR, et al. Requirement for RORgamma in thymocyte survival and lymphoid organ development. Science. 2000;288:2369–73.

77. Hirahara K, Ghoreschi K, Laurence A, Yang XP, Kanno Y, O'Shea JJ. Signal transduction pathways and transcriptional regulation in Th17 cell differentiation. Cytokine Growth Factor Rev. 2010;21:425–34.

78. Ivanov II, Zhou L, Littman DR. Transcriptional regulation of Th17 cell differentiation. Semin Immunol. 2007;19:409–17.

79. Chu CQ, Mello A, Gulko P, Elkon KB. RORγt overexpression predisposes to increased susceptibility and severity of experimental arthritis. Arthritis Rheum. 2008;58:S936.

80. Yang XO, Pappu BP, Nurieva R, et al. T helper 17 lineage differentiation is programmed by orphan nuclear receptors ROR alpha and ROR gamma. Immunity. 2008;28:29–39.

81. Wheeler R, Trifonova V, Vrbanac E, et al. Inhibition of HIV transmission in human cervicovaginal explants and humanized mice using CD4 aptamer-siRNA chimeras. J Clin Invest. 2011;121:2401–12.

82. Mathur AN, Chang HC, Zisoulis DG, et al. Kaplan, Stat3 and Stat4 direct development of IL-17-secreting Th cells. J Immunol. 2007;178:4901–7.

83. Harris TJ, Grosso JF, Yen HR, et al. Cutting edge: an in vivo requirement for STAT3 signaling in TH17 development and TH17-dependent autoimmunity. J Immunol. 2007;179:4313–7.

84. Wei L, Laurence A, Elias KM, O'Shea JJ. IL-21 is produced by Th17 cells and drives IL-17 production in a STAT3-dependent manner. J Biol Chem. 2007;282:34605–10.

85. Chen Z, Laurence A, Kanno Y, et al. Selective regulatory function of Socs3 in the formation of IL-17-secreting T cells. Proc Natl Acad Sci U S A. 2006;103:8137–42.

86. Schraml BU, Hildner K, Ise W, et al. The AP-1 transcription factor Batf controls T(H)17 differentiation. Nature. 2009;460: 405–9.

87. Brustle A, Heink S, Huber M, et al. The development of inflammatory T(H)-17 cells requires interferon-regulatory factor 4. Nat Immunol. 2007;8:958–66.

88. Murphy TL, Tussiwand R, Murphy KM. Specificity through cooperation: BATF-IRF interactions control immune-regulatory networks. Nat Rev Immunol. 2013;13:499–509.

89. Sopel N, Graser A, Mousset S, Finotto S. The transcription factor BATF modulates cytokine-mediated responses in T cells. Cytokine Growth Factor Rev. 2016;30:39–45.

90. Sahoo A, Alekseev A, Tanaka K, et al. Batf is important for IL-4 expression in T follicular helper cells. Nat Commun. 2015;6:7997.

91. Huber M, Lohoff M. IRF4 at the crossroads of effector T-cell fate decision. Eur J Immunol. 2014;44:1886–95.

92. Li R, Spolski W, Liao L, et al. BATF-JUN is critical for IRF4-mediated transcription in T cells. Nature. 2012;490:543–6.

Chapter 4
The Role of IL-17/Th17 Pathway in the Pathogenesis of Autoimmune Inflammatory Diseases

4.1 Rheumatoid Arthritis

Rheumatoid arthritis (RA) is characterized by chronic inflammation of the synovium and cartilage degradation and bone destruction. The initial pathological changes take place in the synovium where there is massive infiltration of inflammatory cells. An increased number of IL-17-producing cells are present in RA synovium and IL-17 in synovial fluid in high levels. The level of IL-17 is correlated with the level of IL-23 [1, 2, 3].

Gene transfer of IL-17A into the joint of collagen-induced arthritis (CIA) promoted arthritis and reproduced the key features of RA, such as massive inflammation, cartilage degradation, and bone erosion [4]. Properties of IL-17A are involved in many aspects of RA pathogenesis including activation of endothelial cells; stimulation of epithelial cells, macrophages, dendritic cells, and fibroblast-like synoviocytes to other inflammatory cytokines; activation of macrophages and dendritic cells to produce matrix metalloproteinases causing cartilage degradation; and stimulation of chondrocytes to produce nitric oxide and stimulation of expression RANKL by osteoblasts causing bone erosion [5]. The pathogenic role of IL-17 is confirmed by therapeutic effect of blocking IL-17 activity in arthritis models [6, 7].

C.-Q. Chu, *Targeting the IL-17 Pathway in Inflammatory Disorders*, DOI 10.1007/978-3-319-28040-0_4,
© Springer International Publishing Switzerland 2017

4.2   Spondyloarthritis

Several lines of evidence support a critical role of the IL-23–IL-17 pathway in ankylosing spondylitis (AS). First, the loss of function of IL-23R *R381Q* gene mutation is associated with protection from AS because of impaired IL-17A production [8]. Conversely, IL-23R variants and other AS-associated genes with known effects on the IL-23 pathway are also identified to be strongly associated with AS [9]. Misfolded human leukocyte antigen (HLA)-B27 can generate endoplasmic reticulum stress that orchestrates the unfolded protein response leading to IL-23 production. Macrophages from AS produce increased levels of IL-23. The number of Th17 cells in AS peripheral blood is increased. Monocyte-derived dendritic cells (DC) from AS patients produce increased levels of IL-23 [10]. IL-23 is also overexpressed in AS spinal facet joints [11].

Spondyloarthritis in animal models of HLA-B27 transgenic rats is associated with CD4+ Th17 cells activation. Ankylosing enthesitis in (BXSBxNZB) F1 mice is associated in IL-17 production by T cells. IL-23 overexpression induces a spondyloarthritis-like disease in B10.RIII mice via RORγt+ CD3+ CD4−CD8− T cells that produce IL-17 and IL-22 [12].

4.3   Psoriasis and Psoriatic Arthritis

Psoriatic arthritis (PsA) is a chronic inflammatory and destructive arthritis associated with psoriasis (PsO). Evidence of IL-17/Th17 pathway association with PsO and PsA is from genetic studies on the presence of IL-17 in disease tissue and animal models. For instance, PsA is associated with single nucleotide polymorphisms (SNPs) in the genes encoding IL-23R and IL-23 [13, 14] and in the gene encoding Act1 (*TRAF3IP2*), the adaptor molecule of IL-17R [15]. These data suggest that the IL-23-mediated IL-17 axis has a central role in the pathogenesis of PsO and PsA. This notion is further supported by elevated expression of IL-23 and IL-23R and IL-17A and IL-17R in psoriatic skin and synovial fluid from patients with PsA [16–19]. In animal models, both IL-23 and IL-17A are shown to induce psoriasis-like skin inflammation. For instance, intradermal injection of IL-23, but not IL-12, induces epidermal hyperplasia with parakeratosis [20]. IL-23-induced psoriasis is IL-17A-dependent [21]. Imiquimod-induced psoriasis-like inflammation of skin exhibits increased expression of IL-23, IL-17A, and IL-17F. Furthermore, IL-17RA deficiency completely abolished the inflammation [22]. In humans with psoriasis, IL-17RA is highly expressed in both lesional and non-lesional skin keratinocytes. In lesional but not non-lesional skin, IL-17A is also overexpressed [23]. It has been shown that IL-17A stimulates keratinocyte expression of CCL20, CXCL1, CXCL2, CXCL3, CXCL5, and CXCL8 (IL-8), which induces recruitment of inflammatory cells including neutrophils into the site of inflammation [24]. CCL20 may directly recruit CCR6+ inflammatory cells including Th17 cells, thereby establishing a positive feedback loop for maintenance of skin inflammation [24].

4.4   Multiple Sclerosis

Experimental autoimmune encephalomyelitis (EAE) is a mouse model of human multiple sclerosis (MS). EAE is commonly used to investigate into the pathogenesis of MS. The essential role of the IL-23 and IL-17/Th17 pathway in the pathogenesis of EAE has been clearly demonstrated in many studies [25, 26] (see above). Elevated levels of IL-23 in blood and cerebral spinal fluid (CSF) have been demonstrated in patients with MS [27, 28]. The elevated level of IL-23 is down-regulated in patients treated with interferon-β, which correlates with clinical improvement suggesting the pathogenic role of IL-23. IL-17A levels are elevated in the blood and central nervous system (CNS) of MS patients, especially during relapse [29–31], and CNS Th17 cells are associated with active disease [32]. It was also shown that human Th17 cells are able to kill neurons and promote CNS inflammation [33].

4.5   Inflammatory Bowel Disease

Crohn's disease is a chronic inflammatory bowel disease, which is also associated with extraintestinal manifestations such as peripheral arthritis and/or axial spondylitis. Genomic data have implicated the IL-23 and IL-17/Th17 pathway in /-17 axis in inflammatory bowel disease in general and Crohn's disease in particular. SNPs in *Il23r* as well as in genes involved in IL-23 and IL-17 regulation have been reported in Crohn's disease [34]. IL-17A-producing CD4+ Th17 cells are increased in both peripheral blood and lamina propria of Crohn's disease [35]. However, conflicting results have been observed in Crohn's disease when IL-23 is blocked or IL-17A and IL-17RA are blocked (see Chap. 5), that is, blockade of IL-23 is beneficial, while blocking IL-17 signaling either provides no benefit or is detrimental to Crohn's disease [36–39].

References

1. Ciofani M, Madar A, Galan C, et al. A validated regulatory network for Th17 cell specification. Cell. 2012;151:289–303.
2. Dang EV, Barbi J, Yang HY, et al. Control of T(H)17/T(reg) balance by hypoxia-inducible factor 1. Cell. 2011;146:772–84.
3. Kotake S, Udagawa N, Takahashi N, et al. IL-17 in synovial fluids from patients with rheumatoid arthritis is a potent stimulator of osteoclastogenesis. J Clin Invest. 1999;103:1345–52.
4. Zrioual S, Toh ML, Tournadre A, et al. IL-17RA and IL-17RC receptors are essential for IL-17 A-induced ELR+ CXC chemokine expression in synoviocytes and are overexpressed in rheumatoid blood. J Immunol. 2008;180:655–63.
5. Chu CQ, Muhkerjee P, Kim DJ, et al. Regulation of IL-17 in rheumatoid arthritis. Arthritis Rheum. 2006;54:4113.
6. Hirahara K, Ghoreschi K, Yang XP, et al. Interleukin-27 priming of T cells controls IL-17 production in trans via induction of the ligand PD-L1. Immunity. 2012;36:1017–30.
7. Lubberts E, Joosten LA, van de Loo FA, Schwarzenberger P, Kolls J, van den Berg WB. Overexpression of IL-17 in the knee joint of collagen type II immunized mice promotes collagen arthritis and aggravates joint destruction. Inflamm Res. 2002;51:102–4.

8. Miossec P, Kolls JK. Targeting IL-17 and TH17 cells in chronic inflammation. Nat Rev Drug Discov. 2012;11:763–76.

9. Lubberts E, Koenders MI, Oppers-Walgreen B, et al. Treatment with a neutralizing anti-murine interleukin-17 antibody after the onset of collagen-induced arthritis reduces joint inflammation, cartilage destruction, and bone erosion. Arthritis Rheum. 2004;50:650–9.

10. Burton PR, Clayton DG, Cardon LR, et al. Association scan of 14,500 nonsynonymous SNPs in four diseases identifies autoimmunity variants. Nat Genet. 2007;39:1329–37.

11. Cortes A, Hadler J, Pointon JP, et al. Identification of multiple risk variants for ankylosing spondylitis through high-density genotyping of immune-related loci. Nat Genet. 2013;45:730–8.

12. Prevosto C, Goodall JC, Hill Gaston JS. Cytokine secretion by pathogen recognition receptor-stimulated dendritic cells in rheumatoid arthritis and ankylosing spondylitis. J Rheumatol. 2012;39:1918–28.

13. Appel H, Maier R, Bleil J, et al. In situ analysis of interleukin-23- and interleukin-12-positive cells in the spine of patients with ankylosing spondylitis. Arthritis Rheum. 2013;65:1522–9.

14. Sherlock JP, Joyce-Shaikh B, Turner SP, et al. IL-23 induces spondyloarthropathy by acting on ROR-gammat+ CD3+CD4-CD8-entheseal resident T cells. Nat Med. 2012;18:1069–76.

15. Bowes J, Orozco G, Flynn E, et al. Confirmation of TNIP1 and IL23A as susceptibility loci for psoriatic arthritis. Ann Rheum Dis. 2011;70:1641–4.

16. Manel N, Unutmaz D, Littman DR. The differentiation of human T(H)-17 cells requires transforming growth factor-beta and induction of the nuclear receptor RORgammat. Nat Immunol. 2008;9:641–9.

17. Filer C, Ho P, Smith RL, et al. Investigation of association of the IL12B and IL23R genes with psoriatic arthritis. Arthritis Rheum. 2008;58:3705–9.

18. Huffmeier U, Uebe S, Ekici AB, et al. Common variants at TRAF3IP2 are associated with susceptibility to psoriatic arthritis and psoriasis. Nat Genet. 2010;42:996–9.

19. Raychaudhuri SP, Raychaudhuri SK, Genovese MC. IL-17 receptor and its functional significance in psoriatic arthritis. Mol Cell Biochem. 2012;359:419–29.

20. Mrabet D, Laadhar L, Sahli H, et al. Synovial fluid and serum levels of IL-17, IL-23, and CCL-20 in rheumatoid arthritis and psoriatic arthritis: a Tunisian cross-sectional study. Rheumatol Int. 2013;33:265–6.

21. Tonel G, Conrad C, Laggner U, et al. Cutting edge: A critical functional role for IL-23 in psoriasis. J Immunol. 2010;185: 5688–91.
22. Chan JR, Blumenschein W, Murphy E, et al. IL-23 stimulates epidermal hyperplasia via TNF and IL-20R2-dependent mechanisms with implications for psoriasis pathogenesis. J Exp Med. 2006;203:2577–87.
23. Rizzo HL, Kagami S, Phillips KG, Kurtz SE, Jacques SL, Blauvelt A. IL-23-mediated psoriasis-like epidermal hyperplasia is dependent on IL-17 A. J Immunol. 2011;186:1495–502.
24. van der Fits L, Mourits S, Voerman JS, et al. Imiquimod-induced psoriasis-like skin inflammation in mice is mediated via the IL-23/IL-17 axis. J Immunol. 2009;182:5836–45.
25. Infante-Duarte C, Horton HF, Byrne MC, Kamradt T. Microbial lipopeptides induce the production of IL-17 in Th cells. J Immunol. 2000;165:6107–15.
26. Aggarwal S, Ghilardi N, Xie MH, de Sauvage FJ, Gurney AL. Interleukin-23 promotes a distinct CD4 T cell activation state characterized by the production of interleukin-17. J Biol Chem. 2003;278:1910–4.
27. Johansen C, Usher PA, Kjellerup RB, Lundsgaard D, Iversen L, Kragballe K. Characterization of the interleukin-17 isoforms and receptors in lesional psoriatic skin. Br J Dermatol. 2009; 160:319–24.
28. Harper EG, Guo C, Rizzo H, et al. Th17 cytokines stimulate CCL20 expression in keratinocytes in vitro and in vivo: implications for psoriasis pathogenesis. J Invest Dermatol. 2009;129: 2175–83.
29. Krakauer M, Sorensen P, Khademi M, Olsson T, Sellebjerg F. Increased IL-10 mRNA and IL-23 mRNA expression in multiple sclerosis: interferon-beta treatment increases IL-10 mRNA expression while reducing IL-23 mRNA expression. Mult Scler. 2008;14:622–30.
30. Alexander JS, Harris MK, Wells SR, et al. Alterations in serum MMP-8, MMP-9, IL-12p40 and IL-23 in multiple sclerosis patients treated with interferon-beta1b. Mult Scler. 2010;16: 801–9.
31. Matusevicius D, Kivisakk P, He B, et al. Interleukin-17 mRNA expression in blood and CSF mononuclear cells is augmented in multiple sclerosis. Mult Scler. 1999;5:101–4.
32. Durelli L, Conti L, Clerico M, et al. T-helper 17 cells expand in multiple sclerosis and are inhibited by interferon-beta. Ann Neurol. 2009;65:499–509.

33. Brucklacher-Waldert V, Stuerner K, Kolster M, Wolthausen J, Tolosa E. Phenotypical and functional characterization of T helper 17 cells in multiple sclerosis. Brain. 2009;132:3329–41.

34. Tzartos JS, Friese MA, Craner MJ. Interleukin-17 production in central nervous system-infiltrating T cells and glial cells is associated with active disease in multiple sclerosis. Am J Pathol. 2008;172:146–55.

35. Kebir H, Kreymborg K, Ifergan I. A. et al. Human TH17 lymphocytes promote blood-brain barrier disruption and central nervous system inflammation. Nat Med. 2007;13:1173–5.

36. Duerr RH, Taylor KD, Brant SR, et al. A genome-wide association study identifies IL23R as an inflammatory bowel disease gene. Science. 2006;314:1461–3.

37. Kobayashi T, Okamoto S, Hisamatsu T, et al. IL23 differentially regulates the Th1/Th17 balance in ulcerative colitis and Crohn's disease. Gut. 2008;57:1682–9.

38. Sandborn WJ, Feagan BG, Fedorak RN, et al. A randomized trial of Ustekinumab, a human interleukin-12/23 monoclonal antibody, in patients with moderate-to-severe Crohn's disease. Gastroenterology. 2008;135:1130–41.

39. Sandborn WJ, Gasink C, Gao LL, et al. Ustekinumab induction and maintenance therapy in refractory Crohn's disease. N Engl J Med. 2012;367:1519–28.

Chapter 5
Therapeutic Applications: Strategies and Molecules Targeting the IL-17/Th17 Pathway

As shown in Fig. 5.1a–e, there are multiple points where the interleukin 17 (IL-17)/Th17 pathway can be blocked for therapy of inflammatory diseases. These include targeting cytokines that promote Th17 cells, targeting IL-17 cytokines, targeting IL-17Rs, targeting Th17 master transcription factor RAR-related orphan receptor gamma t (RORγt), and blocking IL-17 cytokine signaling. Currently clinically available agents and those in late-phase development blocking IL-17 pathway are almost exclusively monoclonal antibodies. Small molecules blocking RORγt activity appear to be promising, and several molecules are in early-phase trials. RNAi offers precise blockade of the target but delivery of efficient quantity for therapeutic purpose is a challenge. More research on this aspect is required before it can be tested clinically.

5.1 Targeting Upper Stream Cytokines

5.1.1 Impact on IL-17/Th17 Cells by Blocking Interleukin 6 and Tumor Necrosis Factor Signaling

Several inflammatory cytokines including IL-6, IL-1, and tumor necrosis factor (TNF) are indicated to induce Th17 cell

C.-Q. Chu, *Targeting the IL-17 Pathway in Inflammatory Disorders*, DOI 10.1007/978-3-319-28040-0_5,
© Springer International Publishing Switzerland 2017

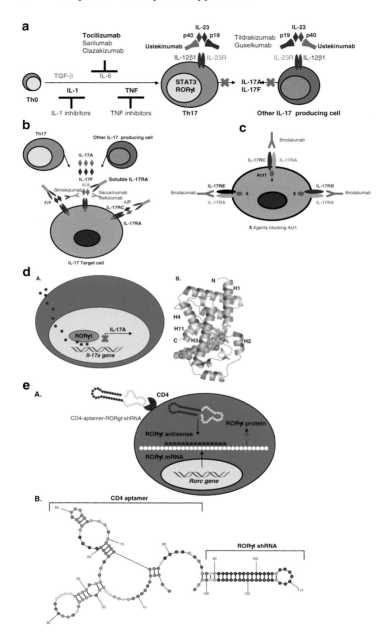

FIGURE 5.1 (**a**) Agents blocking Th17 cell upper stream cytokines. IL-6, TNF, and IL-1 are all shown to involve Th17 cell differentiation. In particular, IL-6 has been shown to be an essential inflammatory cytokine in initiation of Th17 cell differentiation. Biological agents blocking TNF, IL-6, or IL-1 are efficacious therapeutics and may suppress Th17 cells in vivo. Monoclonal antibodies to the IL-12/IL-23 shared subunit, p40 (ustekinumab), and to IL-23-specific subunit, p19 (tildrakizumab and guselkumab), have been developed and demonstrated highly efficacious in treating inflammatory diseases which are mediated by IL-17/Th17 pathway. (**b**) Agents blocking IL-17 cytokine activities. Secukinumab and ixekizumab are two monoclonal antibodies to IL-17A, which have been approved for treating inflammatory diseases and are highly efficacious for psoriasis. They may also interfere with IL-17A/F activity. An IL-17A and IL-17F bispecific antibody, bimekizumab, is under early-phase clinical investigation. A soluble IL-17R fused with IgG Fc can be developed as a therapeutic agent to block IL-17 binging to the receptors. (**c**) Inhibitors blocking IL-17 signaling. Brodalumab is a human monoclonal antibody to IL-17RA, which is effective for psoriasis and psoriatic arthritis (see Fig. 5.2b). Since IL-17RA is a common receptor for IL-17A, IL-17F, IL-17E (IL-25), and IL-17C, the effect of brodalumab may be broad and undesired outcome may be expected. Agents blocking Act1 may also have broad suppressive effect. (**d**) Small molecule drugs blocking RORγ activity. (A) Several small molecules have been identified to block RORγ/RORγt activity. Three such small molecule drugs are in Phase I clinical studies. (**b**) Digoxin is a prototype small molecule that is able to inhibit RORγt activity and suppress Th17 development. Schematic representation of ligand-binding domain of RORγt (*dark blue*) bound with digoxin. Bound digoxin is depicted with carbon atoms in cyan and oxygen atoms in red (Reproduced with permission from © The American Society for Biochemistry and Molecular Biology. All rights reserved. Fujita-Sato et al. [1]). (**e**) Small interference RNA suppressing RORγt. Schematic graph shows shRNA to RORγt is delivered by CD4 aptamer into Th17 cell. (**a**) An RNA aptamer specific for CD4 is linked with RORγt shRNA to form a chimeric molecule. In the cytoplasm, RORγt antisense is released and binds to and degrades RORγt mRNA to prevent the protein translation. (**b**) Predicted secondary structure of CD4 aptamer and RORγt shRNA chimera (Reproduced with permission from © Elsevier. All rights reserved. Song et al. [2]). *IL* interleukin, *RAR* related orphan receptor gamma *t* RORγt, *TNF* tumor necrosis factor

differentiation in in vitro experiments. Blocking these cytokine activities has been in practice for treating inflammatory diseases before the identification of Th17 cells. In theory, blocking TNF, IL-1, and IL-6 treatment will have a negative effect on Th17 cell development. Indeed, clinical observations suggest that inhibition of IL-6 signaling and blocking TNF activity has an impact on Th17 cells. For example, it was reported that TNF is able to promote Th17 cells in rheumatoid arthritis (RA) patients [3] and treatment with anti-TNF in patients who showed an adequate response had a decreased number of Th17 cells in the circulation [4, 5]. Paradoxically, patients treated with anti-TNF but had inadequate response have exhibited an increased number of Th17 cells (see below) [5–8]. IL-6 is the major cytokine that has been well established in induction of Th17 cells (see above), and IL-6 was required for regulatory T cells (Tregs) to convert to Th17 cells in the arthritis model [9]. The therapeutic efficacy of blocking IL-6 signaling in RA is also firmly established. Indeed, targeting IL-6 in early RA results in decreased Th17 cells [10, 11].

Tocilizumab is a humanized monoclonal antibody against both membrane and soluble IL-6Rα. Tocilizumab is approved to treat RA and juvenile idiopathic arthritis. Previous case series and pilot studies suggested therapeutic efficacy of tocilizumab in spondyloarthritis and psoriatic arthritis (PsA). However, the recently conducted BUILDER-1 and BUILDER-2 prospective randomized, placebo-controlled trials did not confirm the previous findings in TNF inhibitor-naive and TNF inhibitor-refractory ankylosing spondylitis, even though the IL-6 signaling blockade was effective, which has been demonstrated by the reduction of acute-phase reactants [12]. Furthermore, sarilumab, another monoclonal antibody against IL-6Rα also failed to show efficacy in TNF inhibitor-naive ankylosing spondylitis patients [13].

A humanized anti-IL-6 monoclonal antibody clazakizumab, which had promising results in patients with moderate-to-severe RA, was also recently found to be moderately effective in PsA in Phase IIb clinical trial with a clear response in musculoskeletal disease manifestations (arthritis, enthesitis, and dactylitis) [14]. Interestingly, there is only limited response in skin psoriasis, with a maximal PSAI75 response for clazakizumab at 28 % versus 12.2 % for placebo [14]. This response rate is much lower than those blocking IL-23 or IL-17 cytokines (Fig. 5.2a, b). The less robust response of IL-6 signaling blockade in treating psoriasis may be in line with the notion that in vivo pathogenic Th17 cells are dependent on IL-23; IL-6-dependent Th17 cells are more

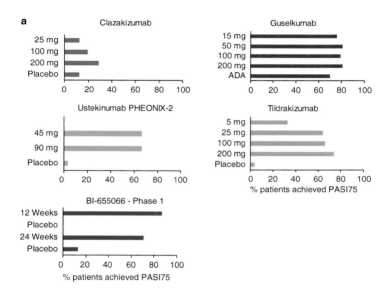

FIGURE 5.2 (**a, b**) Efficacy of monoclonal antibodies targeting IL-17/Th17 pathway in psoriasis. Graphs show the percentage of psoriasis patients that achieved PASI 75 in each individual clinical study, and they are not head-to-head comparison studies. (**a**) Clazakizumab is a humanized monoclonal antibody to IL-6. Ustekinumab is a humanized monoclonal antibody to IL-12/IL-23 shared p40 subunit. BI-655066 is a human and guselkumab are humanized monoclonal antibodies to IL-23 p19 subunit. (**b**) Secukinumab is a human and ixekizumab is a humanized monoclonal antibody to IL-17A. Brodalumab is a human monoclonal antibody to IL-17RA. *IL* interleukin, *PASI 75* 75 % improvement of Psoriasis Area Severity Index

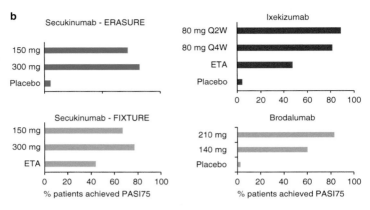

FIGURE 5.2 (continued)

important in host defense in immunity against pathogens and less pathogenic in autoimmune inflammatory diseases [15].

5.1.2   Blocking IL-23

Given its critical role in the development of Th17 cells, naturally IL-23 is an attractive target. Several monoclonal antibodies are being developed to neutralize IL-23 activity.

5.1.2.1   Monoclonal Antibodies Against IL-12 and IL-23 Shared p40 Subunit

Two monoclonal antibodies have been developed to target the shared p40 subunit of IL-12 and IL-23, namely, ustekinumab and briakinumab.

Ustekinumab

Ustekinumab in Psoriasis

Ustekinumab is initially developed to target IL-12 activity before the discovery of IL-23. This fully human IgG1 monoclonal antibody binds to the shared p40 subunit of IL-12 and

IL-23 and blocks its binding to the IL-12Rβ1 receptor protein on the surface of the immune cell, thereby inhibiting the bioactivity of both IL-12 and IL-23 [16]. Ustekinumab interferes with development of Th1 and Th17 cells and also keratinocyte activation. Ustekinumab was approved for the treatment of moderate-to-severe plaque psoriasis by the European Medicines Agency (EMA) in 2008 and US Food and Drug Administration (FDA) in 2009 and active PsA jointly by EMA and FDA in 2013 in cases of inadequate response to disease-modifying antirheumatic drugs (DMARDs) or alternative to anti-TNF [16]. Data from clinical trials and post-market registries indicate that ustekinumab is a safe and efficacious agent in treating moderate-to-severe plaque psoriasis. In two Phase III parallel double-blind placebo controlled studies (PHOENIX-1 and PHOENIX-2), ustekinumab was administered by subcutaneous injection at 45 and 90 mg every 12 weeks. A 75 % reduction in the Psoriasis Area Severity Index score (PASI 75) was achieved in 66.7–67.1 % of patients taking 45 mg dose and 66.4–75.7 % of patients taking 90 mg while in only 3.1–3.7 % of those taking placebo at 12 weeks [17, 18]. In a randomized comparative study, ustekinumab at both 45 mg and 90 mg doses was shown to be more effective than etanercept at 50 mg twice a week [19] (Fig. 5.2a).

Ustekinumab in PsA

Ustekinumab is also approved for treating adult patients with active PsA who failed methotrexate and/or TNF inhibitors. In a Phase III trial (PSUMMIT-1), 615 patients who were naive to biological therapies were treated with ustekinumab at 45 mg or 90 mg. At week 24, 42.4 % patients treated with 45 mg and 49.5 % treated with 90 mg of ustekinumab achieved the primary end point of an American College of Rheumatology response (ACR20) versus 22.8 % with placebo ($p < 0.001$ for both comparisons). There were also significant differences between ustekinumab- and placebo-treated groups for ACR50 and ACR70 responses [20]. In the PSUMMIT-2 trial, 312 psoriatic arthritis patients with active disease including those failed TNF inhibitors were treated with ustekinumab. Similar to the findings in PSUMMIT-1, at week 24, the ACR20 response rate was significantly higher in both ustekinumab arms (45 or 90 mg) than placebo regardless of their prior treatment agents. PSUMMIT-2 clearly demonstrates that ustekinumab is a valid therapy for PsA patients who have failed to respond to TNF inhibitors. However, these TNF inhibitor-experienced patients seemed to achieve a less robust response than TNF inhibitor-naive patients. That is, among patients who failed prior TNF inhibitors, only 36.7 % (ustekinumab 45 mg) and 34.5 % (ustekinumab 90 mg) achieved ACR20 response compared with 14.5 % in the placebo-treated group [21]. Ustekinumab slows down radiographic progression in PsA and is also effective for enthesitis and dactylitis [20, 21].

Long-term safety of ustekinumab has been proven in the 5-year extension of two major clinical trials. There are no increased adverse events and no positive or negative effects in cardiovascular outcomes after five continuous years of follow-up [22, 23]. Data from over 12,000 patients in several registries show no increased risk of malignancy, major adverse cardiovascular events, serious infections, or mortality [24–26].

Ustekinumab in Crohn's Disease

In a small Phase II trial (https://clinicaltrials.gov/ NCT00265122) [27], ustekinumab seemed effective at inducing a clinical response at weeks 4 and 6, but not at week 8. Interestingly, a better clinical response was seen in patients who had previously failed TNF inhibitors, for example, in a larger Phase IIb trial (CERTIFI, https://clinicaltrials.gov/ NCT00771667) including patients with moderate-to-severe disease who failed previous TNF inhibitors [28]. Ustekinumab was given as an intravenous (IV) infusion at 1, 3, or 6 mg/kg at week 0 for induction therapy. At week 6, Crohn's Disease Activity Index (CDAI) response was 37 %, 34 %, and 40 % for 1, 3, and 6 mg/kg of ustekinumab, respectively, compared with 23.5 % for placebo ($p = 0.02, 0.06$, and 0.005). However, rates of remission in ustekinumab-treated groups were not significantly different from those that were placebo-treated. During the maintenance phase, the 145 responders at week 6 were re-randomized to receive either placebo or subcutaneous ustekinumab 90 mg at weeks 8 and 16. At week 22, the ustekinumab-treated group achieved a higher response rate than the placebo group (69 % versus 42.5 %, $p < 0.001$) and a higher remission rate (42 % versus 27 %, $p < 0.03$). These results indicate that blocking the shared subunit p40 of IL-12 and IL-23 by ustekinumab is beneficial in those patients with Crohn's disease who failed TNF inhibitors. Three Phase III trials (https://clinicaltrials.gov/NCT01369329; NCT01369342; NCT01369355) are ongoing to further evaluate the safety and efficacy of ustekinumab in treating moderate-to-severe Crohn's disease.

It is conceivable that ustekinumab may interfere with both IL-12 and IL-23 signaling and subsequently affect both Th1 and Th17 cells and their cytokines. However, downregulation of p40 and IL-23p19, but not IL-12p35, in psoriatic skin lesions was observed in ustekinumab-treated patients suggesting that interference with IL-23 rather than IL-12 activity is responsible for this clinical improvement [29]. This is in concordance with results of studies in murine experimental autoimmune encephalomyelitis (EAE) and collagen-induced arthritis (CIA), which have indicated that IL-23 rather than IL-12 is responsible for the chronic inflammation [30]. Investigations into expression of Th17 versus Th1 cell cytokines in ustekinumab-treated patients will be required to further verify the exact mechanism of ustekinumab action in vivo.

Ustekinumab in Multiple Sclerosis

Safety and efficacy of ustekinumab was also evaluated in treating in relapsing-remitting multiple sclerosis (https://clinicaltrials.gov/NCT00207727). Contrary to the high expectation, ustekinumab failed to provide improvement in magnetic resonance imaging (MRI) lesions in patients with relapsing-remitting multiple sclerosis [31], in spite of the strong evidence to support the role of IL-23 and Th17 in EAE.

Briakinumab

Briakinumab is another fully human antibody against the IL-12 and IL-23 shared p40 subunit. Unfortunately it was withdrawn from the market due to the safety concerns of major cardiac events in patients treated with briakinumab. The available data from clinical trials showed that it was a potent agent in treating psoriasis, PsA, and Crohn's disease [32–36]. Nevertheless, the clinical efficacy of briakinumab in these diseases provided further evidence to prove the importance of IL-23 signaling in these conditions.

5.1.2.2   Monoclonal Antibodies Against IL-23 p19

Various IL-23 p19-specific monoclonal antibodies are currently undergoing clinical development. Specifically targeting the p19 subunit of IL-23 is advantageous because it spares the IL-12-mediated Th1 response [37]. In addition to preservation of Th1 host immunity against infections, it has been stipulated that the intact Th1 pathway may actually contribute to inhibition of Th17 cells. Thus, it has been hypothesized that targeting the p19 subunit of IL-23 may be as effective but safer than blocking p40.

Tildrakizumab

Tildrakizumab is a humanized monoclonal antibody (IgG1k) against IL-23 p19 subunit. In a randomized, double-blind, Phase IIb clinical trial, tildrakizumab was effective in treating patients with moderate-to-severe plaque psoriasis (Fig. 5.2a). At week 16, a significantly higher proportion of patients treated with tildrakizumab achieved PASI 75 at all doses compared with placebo [38]. In a Phase I trial [39], the main cellular source of IL-23 in the lesional skin was identified to be CD11c+ myeloid dendritic cells, CD15+ neutrophils, and

CD163+ macrophages. The number of CD4+ and CD8+ T cells in the skin decreased significantly after tildrakizumab treatment. CD4+ Th17 cells expressing CCR6 binds to CCL20, which is overexpressed in lesional skin in psoriasis. Tildrakizumab significantly reduced CCL20 expression. This is consistent with the reduction of CD4+ T cells [39]. Unfortunately, due to technology limitations, the study did not directly examine the expression of Th17 cells and their cytokines, but this is planned for investigation in subsequent Phase III trials. Two Phase III clinical trials are ongoing for moderate-to-severe plaque psoriasis (https://clinicaltrials. gov/NCT01729754; NCT01722331).

BI-655066

BI-655066 is a high-affinity monoclonal antibody against the p19 subunit of IL-23. Clinical efficacy was demonstrated in psoriasis in a Phase I trial. After a single dose, PASI 75 was achieved in 87 %, PASI 90 in 58 %, and PASI 100 in 16 % of subjects (Fig. 5.2a) [40]. The most common side effects were mild-to-moderate upper respiratory infections including mild nasopharyngitis and mild-to-moderate headache. BI-655066 treatment resulted in significant reductions relative to placebo in the expression of 192 genes identified in skin biopsy specimens including those in the IL-23/IL-17 pathway related [40]. A dose-ranging Phase II trial in psoriasis in comparison with ustekinumab has been completed, and data publication is pending (https://clinicaltrials.gov/ NCT02054481). Several Phase II clinical trials are ongoing to treat moderate-to-severe Crohn's disease (https://clinicaltrials.gov/NCT02031276), in ankylosing spondylitis (https:// clinicaltrials.gov/NCT02047110), and in severe persistent asthma (https://clinicaltrials.gov/NCT02443298). Two Phase III trials in moderate-to-severe plaque psoriasis to compare BI-655066 with ustekinumab are ongoing (https://clinicaltrials.gov/NCT02684357; NCT02684370) as well as one Phase III study in moderate-to-severe plaque psoriasis comparing BI-655066 with adalimumab (https://clinicaltrials.gov/ NCT02694523).

Guselkumab

Guselkumab is a fully human IgG1k monoclonal antibody against p19 subunit of IL-23. In a Phase II clinical trial, patients with moderate-to-severe psoriasis were treated with guselkumab versus adalimumab. Guselkumab-treated patient were significantly more likely to achieve a physician global assessment (PGA) score of 0 (clear of plaque psoriasis) or 1 (almost clear of plaque psoriasis) when compared with placebo. At week 16, a score of 0 or 1 on the PGA was seen in 58 % of patients randomized to adalimumab, which was significantly lower than that achieved by patients on 50, 100, and 200 mg doses of guselkumab: 79 %, 86 %, and 83 %, respectively ($p < 0.05$ for all comparisons); while 7 % was achieved in the placebo group. Treatment response assessment by PASI 75 also demonstrated that guselkumab is superior to adalimumab (Fig. 5.2a). While 70 % of patients treated with adalimumab achieved PASI 75 response, in guselkumab-treated patients, 76 % in the 15 mg, 81 % in the 50 mg, 79 % in the 100 mg, and 81 % in the 200 mg dose group, respectively, achieved PASI 75 response [41].

In a Phase I trial, guselkumab responders showed significant reductions of the Th17 pathway gene expression in lesional skin and serum IL-17A levels from baseline at week 1 ($p = 0.031$) and week 12 ($p = 0.0015$), while there were no significant changes in Th1 cytokines [42]. These data indicate the critical role of IL-23 and the downstream Th17 pathway in the pathogenesis of psoriasis. Three Phase III trials are ongoing to further investigate the therapeutic efficacy in psoriasis (https://clinicaltrials.gov/NCT02207244; NCT02207231; NCT02203032).

5.2   Targeting Th17 Cytokines

Secukinumab and ixekizumab are two monoclonal antibodies, which have already been approved for clinical applications.

5.2.1 Secukinumab

Secukinumab in Psoriasis

Secukinumab is a fully human IgG1k monoclonal antibody against IL-17A [43]. It was first approved in Japan in 2014 for treating psoriasis and PsA and in the USA and in Europe as a first-line drug for the treatment of moderate-to-severe plaque psoriasis in 2015 and later also approved for the treatment of PsA and ankylosing spondylitis.

The therapeutic effect of secukinumab was first demonstrated in three proof-of-concept studies in three different diseases, psoriasis, RA, and uveitis [44]. The most remarkable effect is in patients with psoriasis. A single dose of 3 mg/kg secukinumab was able to reduce the disease severity by 58 % relative to baseline compared with 4 % reduction in placebo-treated patients. The therapeutic effect lasted for 12 weeks. Secukinumab treatment led to the decrease of CD3$^+$ T cells and IL-17A expressing cells in the skin. Decreased gene expression was also observed for IL-17F, IL-21, IL-22, shared p40 subunit of IL-12 and IL-23, TNF, IL-6, and CCL20 [44]. The suppressive effect of secukinumab on both downstream and upper stream cytokines of Th17 cells suggests that IL-17A may act on a positive feedback loop to further promote Th17 cell differentiation.

In later clinical trial phases for treating psoriasis, secukinumab was administered with initial intravenous or subcutaneous loading doses at baseline, weeks 1, 2, 3, and 4, followed by subcutaneous administration every 4 weeks. Four Phase III trials were conducted in plaque psoriasis (ERASURE, https://clinicaltrials.gov/NCT01365455; FIXTURE, NCT01358578; FEATURE, NCT01555125; JUNCTURE, NCT01636687). Across the trials, the co-primary end points were the response rates at week 12 based on PASI 75 and Investigator's Global Assessment (IGA) scale (proportion of patients with a score of 0–1 plus a reduction of ≥ 2 points from baseline). This IGA scale is a more robust assessment with 0 being clear and 1 almost clear [45]. Secukinumab was administered in 150 and 300 mg. In the

ERASURE trial, the PASI 75 response rates were 72 % and 82 % in the secukinumab 150 and 300 mg doses, respectively, compared with 5 % in the placebo group (Fig. 5.2b) [43], and the IGA response rates were 51 % and 65 % versus 2 %, respectively. In the FIXTURE trial, secukinumab was compared with etanercept. Secukinumab at both 150 mg and 300 mg doses achieved significantly higher response rates than etanercept, that is, PASI 75 was 67 % and 77 % for secukinumab 150 mg and 300 mg, respectively, versus 44 % for etanercept ($p < 0.001$ comparing both secukinumab groups versus etanercept). The IGA response rates in the corresponding treatment groups were 51 %, 63 %, and 27 %, respectively ($p < 0.001$ comparing both secukinumab groups vs etanercept) [43]. Similar positive results in favor of secukinumab were also observed in the FEATURE [46] and JUNCTURE [47] trials. Across all the trials, maintenance therapy was continued from week 12 to week 52 and efficacy of secukinumab was well maintained.

Secukinumab in PsA

Efficacious treatment of secukinumab for PsA was demonstrated in two Phase III trials (https://clinicaltrials.gov/ NCT01392326 and NCT01752634). PsA patients with active disease who failed DMARDs and/or anti-TNF were included [48, 49]. In the FUTURE 1 trial, patients were treated with secukinumab 10 mg/kg intravenously at weeks 0, 2, and 4 followed by 75 or 150 mg subcutaneously every 4 weeks [48]. ACR20 response at week 24 was 51 % and 50 %, respectively, for secukinumab 75 and 150 mg groups compared with 17 % in placebo group. Secukinumab at both doses was also effective for treating dactylitis and inhibiting radiographic structural joint damage. The therapeutic effect was maintained throughout 52 weeks [48]. In the FUTURE 2 trial, patients were treated with secukinumab with loading dose at 75, 150, or 300 mg weekly for 5 weeks and then every 4 weeks. An ACR20 response at week 24 was in achieved in 29 %, 51 %, and 54 % for three doses of secukinumab compared with 15 % in the placebo group [49].

Secukinumab in Ankylosing Spondylitis

For ankylosing spondylitis, secukinumab was tested in two Phase III trials, MEASURE 1 (https://clinicaltrials.gov/NCT01358175) and MEASURE 2 (https://clinicaltrials.gov/NCT01649375) [50]. All patients with ankylosing spondylitis had active disease despite treatment with nonsteroidal anti-inflammatory drugs (NSAIDs), and a proportion of patients had failed anti-TNF and/or DMARDs. In the MEASURE 1 trial, secukinumab was loaded by intravenous infusion at 10 mg/kg at week 0, 2, and 4, while in the MEASURE 2 trial, secukinumab was loaded by subcutaneous injection weekly for 4 weeks. Maintenance therapy was administered by subcutaneous injection every 4 weeks at either 75 or 150 mg. At week 16, in the MEASURE 1 trial, the Assessment of Spondyloarthritis International Society response criteria (ASAS20) response rates were 60 % and 61 % for secukinumab at doses of 75 mg and 150 mg, respectively, versus 29 % for placebo ($p < 0.001$ for both comparisons with placebo); in the MEASURE 2 trial, the ASAS20 response rates were 41 % and 61 % for secukinumab at 75 mg and 150 mg, respectively, versus 28 % for placebo ($p = 0.1$ for the 75 mg group; $p < 0.001$ for the 150 mg group). The improvement was sustained throughout 52 weeks. These results indicate that secukinumab at 150 mg subcutaneous dose with either subcutaneous or intravenous loading is efficacious in treating ankylosing spondylitis [50].

Secukinumab in RA

The therapeutic efficacy of secukinumab in RA was evaluated in a Phase II trial with dose-finding regimens (https://clinicaltrials.gov/NCT00928512). Patients were allowed to have concomitant medications including methotrexate between 7.5 and 25 mg/week and/or prednisone ≤10 mg/day. Patients failed DMARD and/or biological agents had a washout period before randomization. Patients were randomized to receive a monthly subcutaneous injection of 25 mg, 75 mg, 150 mg, and 300 mg or placebo [51]. At week 16, the primary end point was not met. At the dose-escalating phase of the study, patients achieving an ACR20 response continued on the same dose, while nonresponders taking 25 and 75 mg doses were increased to 150 mg; nonresponders taking 150 mg were increased to 300 mg, patients taking 300 mg of secukinumab continued the same dose regardless of their response, and those on placebo were given 150 mg of secukinumab. Responders who kept taking 150 mg of secukinumab had the greatest improvement in response over time with 55 % and 40 % of patients achieving an ACR50 and ACR70 response, respectively, at week 52. Among patients taking the placebo who had achieved an ACR20 response by week 16 and were reassigned to 150 mg of secukinumab at week 20, 50 % achieved an ACR50 response and 22.2 % achieved an ACR70 response by week 52 [52]. In another Phase II trial (https://clinicaltrials.gov/NCT01359943), secukinumab was given as a loading dose with either IV infusion at 10 mg/kg at baseline, weeks 2 and 4, from week 8, 150 mg subcutaneous injection every 4 weeks through to week 48, or secukinumab 150 mg subcutaneous injection loading at baseline, weeks 1, 2, 3, and 4 and then followed by every 4 weeks starting at week 8 through to 48 weeks [53]. No difference was observed between the two loading regimens in terms of the efficacy of secukinumab in achieving rates of ACR20 response at week 16. It was demonstrated that secukinumab improved efficacy in reducing disease activity over placebo as measured by the disease activity score 28 (DAS28) and other secondary end points although the primary end point (ACR20) was not met [53].

Another Phase II trial (https://clinicaltrials.gov/NCT01426789) was designed to identify a biomarker to guide treatment response to secukinumab [54]. Secukinumab induced rapid and significant changes from baseline in DAS28-C-reactive protein (CRP) and in ACR20 and ACR50 response rates compared with placebo. However, human leukocyte antigen (HLA)-DRB1* alleles was not able to predict secukinumab response [54].

Patients who did not respond to TNF inhibitors showed increased Th17 cells and IL-23 expression [5, 6]. It would be particularly interesting to delineate whether those patients who had a good response to secukinumab had previously failed TNF inhibitors. In a Phase II trial (https://clinicaltrials.gov/NCT00928512) [51, 52], up to 22.2 % of patients who had previously been exposed to biologics were included, but the size of the subgroup was too small to allow for meaningful subanalysis. It is hypothesized that in the following Phase III trials, those patients who have had an inadequate response to TNF inhibitors should have a good response to secukinumab. The four Phase III trials (REASSURE, https://clinicaltrials.gov/NCT01377012; NURTURE 1, NCT01350804; REASSURE2, NCT01770379; REASSURE-E, NCT01901900]) are designed to treat all RA patients who have had an inadequate response to TNF inhibitors.

Secukinumab in Crohn's Disease

Secukinumab was also trialed in patients with moderate-to-severe Crohn's disease (https://clinicaltrials.gov/NCT01009281) [55]. In this Phase IIa study, secukinumab was administered as an IV infusion at 10 mg/kg on day 1 and day 22. Safety and efficacy were assessed by the Crohn's Disease Activity Index. In the secukinumab-treated group, 21 % discontinued treatment prematurely due to insufficient therapeutic effect compared with 10 % in placebo-treated group. A higher rate of adverse effect was also observed in the secukinumab-treated group including local fungal infections. This study demonstrates that secukinumab was not only ineffective in treating active Crohn's disease but also seemed to be detrimental as was evident by increased adverse effects compared with placebo. Animal models of inflammatory bowel disease and genome-wide association studies clearly suggest an important pathogenic role of IL-17A in perpetuating chronic inflammation by activated T cells [56]. However, results from animals of intestinal inflammation suggested protective roles of IL-17A in T cell-dependent and T cell-independent models of colitis [57, 58].

Secukinumab in Multiple Sclerosis

Secukinumab was tested for multiple sclerosis in a Phase II study (https://clinicaltrials.gov/NCT01051817). Secukinumab reduced the number of new MRI lesions by 63 % compared with placebo-treated patients and saw a trend in reducing annualized relapse rate [59]. Another small Phase II trial (https://clinicaltrials.gov/NCT01433250) to evaluate the safety was completed, but there is no result available. A larger Phase II study (https://clinicaltrials.gov/NCT01874340) was terminated early based on development of another anti-IL-17 fully human monoclonal antibody with better potential for treating multiple sclerosis.

5.2.2   Ixekizumab

Ixekizumab in Psoriasis

Ixekizumab is a humanized, hinge-modified IgG4 monoclonal antibody binding with high affinity to human IL-17A. Ixekizumab is approved by the US FDA for adults with moderate-to-severe plaque psoriasis (http://www.fda.gov/NewsEvents/Newsroom/PressAnnouncements/ucm491872.htm). The efficacy and safety of ixekizumab in treating plaque psoriasis was demonstrated in a Phase II and three Phase III studies, UNCOVER-1 (https://clinicaltrials.gov/NCT01474512), UNCOVER-2 (https://clinicaltrials.gov/NCT01597245), and UNCOVER-3 (https://clinicaltrials.gov/NCT01646177).

These three Phase III trials all had a similar design, and etanercept was compared in UNCOVER-2 and UNCOVER-3 trials [60, 61]. A total of 3866 patients were included in the three trials. Ixekizumab was administered with a loading dose at 160 mg by subcutaneous injection and then followed by 80 mg every 2 weeks or every 4 weeks. All three studies generated similar results. At week 12, ixekizumab demonstrated statistically significant superiority to placebo. The pooled proportion of patients that achieved PASI 75 was 88.7 % and 81.6 % for ixekizumab 80 mg every 2 weeks and 80 mg every 4 weeks, respectively, while this was achieved in only 4.4 % of patients who took placebo ($p < 0.001$ for all groups compared with placebo). PGA (0 or 1) was 81.8 % and 75 % for ixekizumab 80 mg every 2 weeks and 80 mg every 4 weeks, respectively, compared with 3.9 % in the placebo group. These studies showed that ixekizumab was superior to etanercept (50 mg twice weekly). The pooled PASI 75 for the etanercept-treated groups was 47.5 % ($p < 0.0001$, comparing ixekizumab with etanercept groups) (Fig. 5.2b). The pooled PGA (0 or 1) for etanercept was 38.5 % [60, 61].

Ixekizumab in PsA

Efficacy and safety of ixekizumab in treating patients with PsA has been tested in a Phase III study. During the 24-week, SPIRIT-P1 (https://clinicaltrials.gov/NCT01695239) trial, patients who were naive to biologic DMARDs were treated with a 160 mg loading dose followed by 80 mg every 2 weeks or 4 weeks. Both dosage regimens achieved an ACR20 response that was statistically superior to placebo. At 24 weeks, 62 % of patients treated with 80 mg every 2 weeks and 58 % of patients treated with 80 mg every 4 weeks achieved ACR20 response, respectively, compared with 30 % in the placebo group. ACR50 response was 47 % and 40 % for 80 mg every 2 weeks and every 4 weeks groups, respectively, compared with 15 % of patients treated with placebo [62]. Patients treated with both dosing regimens also experienced significantly less radiographic progression of structural joint damage than those treated with placebo. Patients treated with ixekizumab experienced significantly improved quality of life, physical function, and work productivity [63].

Ixekizumab in Ankylosing Spondylitis

Ixekizumab is also being tested for ankylosing spondylitis in two Phase III trials in biologic-naive patients with radiographic axial spondyloarthritis (https://clinicaltrials.gov/NCT02696785) and in patients that are TNF inhibitor-experienced with radiographic axial spondyloarthritis (https://clinicaltrials.gov/NCT02696798).

Ixekizumab in RA

The therapeutic effect of ixekizumab was tested in a Phase I trial in patients with RA by adding it to baseline DMARD therapy [64]. The safety was established in a single-dose treatment regimen. Then the efficacy was demonstrated in regimens where ixekizumab was administered every 2 weeks in various doses. The efficacy was demonstrated by a significant reduction of DAS28 at 10 weeks [64].

The efficacy of ixekizumab in treating RA was first noticed in the proof-of-concept study (https://clinicaltrials.gov/ NCT01236118) [64]. In the Phase II trial (https://clinicaltrials. gov/NCT00966875), the efficacy of ixekizumab in treating active RA was further demonstrated [65, 66]. Both patients who were biologic-naive and had inadequate response to TNF inhibitors were included. Patients who were biologic-naive were treated with a wide range of doses (3, 10, 30, 80, and 180 mg) of ixekizumab every 2 weeks, while patients who had previously had an inadequate response to TNF inhibitors were treated with ixekizumab at 80 mg and 180 mg. At week 12, the primary end point was met in both the biologic-naive and inadequate responder to TNF inhibitor therapy cohorts as measured by rates of ACR20 and ACR50 response and reduction of DAS28-CRP and CDAI. During the long-term observation, the clinical responses observed at week 16 remained the same or improved through to week 64. Further Phase III studies are needed to fully understand the efficacy and safety of long-term treatment with ixekizumab.

5.3   Antibody Against IL-17RA

5.3.1   Brodalumab

Brodalumab in Psoriasis

Brodalumab is a fully human IgG2 monoclonal antibody against IL-17RA. It is known that IL-17A, IL-17A/F, IL-17F, IL-17C, and IL-17E (IL-25) all use IL-17RA for signaling (see Fig. 1.1). The broader target of brodalumab while increasing the potential benefit may also pose a higher risk for more adverse effects. For instance, IL-17E plays a role in Th2-type inflammatory diseases, parasitic infections, and allergic reactions, such as asthma and atopic dermatitis, and promotes eosinophilia in mice. Targeting IL-17RA may interfere with those mechanisms mediated by IL-17E [67]. More data and longer time are required to fully appreciate the pros and cons of blocking the IL-17 receptor versus the ligands.

Brodalumab has been evaluated for therapy in psoriasis and PsA. In a Phase I study conducted in psoriasis patients, a single dose of brodalumab was able to normalize thousands of aberrantly expressed genes in lesional skin within 2 weeks. Interestingly, keratinocyte-expressed genes appeared to be normalized rapidly, whereas T cell-specific gene expression normalization occurred over 6 weeks. These data clearly demonstrated the potency of brodalumab in blocking IL-17RA-mediated signaling [68].

In psoriasis, the effective doses of brodalumab were determined in a Phase II trial [69]. In the Phase III AMAGINE-1 (https://clinicaltrials.gov/NCT01708590) study, at week 12 PASI 75 was achieved in 83.3 % patients treated with brodalumab at 210 mg and 60.3 % at 140 mg compared with 2.7 % in the placebo group. PGA (0–1) was 75.7 % with brodalumab at 210 mg and 53.7 % at 140 mg group compared with 1.4 % in placebo group [70]. In Phase III trials, AMAGINE-2 (https://clinicaltrials.gov/NCT01708603) and AMAGINE-3 (https://clinicaltrials.gov/NCT01708629), patients with moderate-to-severe plaque psoriasis were treated with 140 mg or 210 mg of brodalumab every 2 weeks in comparison with ustekinumab. At 12 weeks, 85–86 % of patients in the brodalumab 210 mg group and 67–69 % in the 140 mg group achieved a PASI 75 compared with 69–70 % in the ustekinumab-treated group as well as 6–8 % in the placebo group [71]. PGA score (0–1) was higher at 79–80 % in the brodalumab 210 mg group and 58–60 % in the 140 mg group compared with 57–61 % and 4 % in the ustekinumab and placebo groups, respectively (Fig. 5.2b) [71].

Brodalumab in PsA

Brodalumab was tested for patients with PsA in a Phase II trial. Patients with active PsA were treated with brodalumab at 140 mg or 280 mg at day 1, week 1, 2, 4, 6, 8, and 10 followed by an open-label extension starting at week 12 with 280 mg every 2 weeks. At week 12, 37 % and 39 % of patients treated with 140 mg and 280 mg of brodalumab, respectively, achieved an ACR20 response compared with 18 % in the placebo group [72].

5.4   Bispecific Antibodies Simultaneously Targeting IL-17 Cytokines and Other Inflammatory Cytokines

In RA, simultaneous blockade of TNF and IL-1 with a combination of etanercept and anakinra resulted in increased rates of serious infections without extra benefit [73]. Similarly, combination therapy with abatacept (blocking T cell co-stimulation) and etanercept also increased the rate of infection in spite of a small therapeutic benefit [74]. Therefore, caution has been taken in designing therapeutic strategies blocking two cytokine activities concomitantly for therapy of inflammatory diseases. However, blocking TNF and IL-17 simultaneously seems to be safe and may achieve a synergistic therapeutic benefit in an animal model of arthritis [6, 75]. Clinically, blocking two cytokine activities at the same time can be achieved by using bispecific therapeutic monoclonal antibodies. Two bispecific antibodies catumaxomab (anti-CD3 and anti-epithelial cell adhesion molecule) and blinatumomab (anti-CD3 and anti-CD19) are approved to treat malignancy [76]. Currently, three bispecific antibodies against IL-17A and IL-17F, three against IL-17A and TNF, and one against IL-23 and IL-17A are under development to treat various autoimmune inflammatory diseases (see Table 5.1). The rationale for blocking TNF and IL-17A is supported by data from observations in patients with RA, ankylosing

TABLE 5.1 Bispecific antibodies inhibiting IL-17 cytokines and other inflammatory cytokines in clinical development

Name	Targets	Diseases	Phase
Bimekizumab	IL-17 A and IL-17F	PsO, PsA, and RA	Phase I
ALX-0761	IL-17 A and IL-17F	PsO	Phase I
RG7624 (NI-1401)	IL-17 A and IL-17F	Inflammatory diseases	Phase I
ABT-122	IL-17 A and TNF	RA, PsA	Phase II
ABBV-257	IL-17 A and TNF	RA	Phase I
COVA322	IL-17 A and TNF	RA, PsA, PsO, AS	Phase II
IL-17/IL-34 biAb	IL-23 and IL-17 A	Inflammatory diseases	Phase I

Data from [76, 79–81]

PsA psoriatic arthritis, *PsO* psoriasis, *RA* rheumatoid arthritis

spondylitis AS, or PsA who were treated with anti-TNF. Interestingly, those patients who had an inadequate response to anti-TNF displayed an increased number of Th17 cells and increased levels of IL-23 [5–8]. These data suggest that the IL-17 pathway is dominated in patients who are not responding to anti-TNF. The hypothesis is that anti-TNF and anti-IL-17 will have a synergistic therapeutic effect. Early-phase clinical studies in RA patients using bispecific antibodies to inhibit both TNF and IL-17 A activities have demonstrated no increased rate of infection [77]. The agent bimekizumab, which blocks both IL-17A and IL-17F, has been tested in a Phase I study to treat patients with psoriasis. A single-dose IV injection demonstrated no serious adverse effects, but clinical meaningful improvement of skin lesions supported the continued development of bimekizumab for treatment of diseases mediated by both IL-17A and IL-17F [78].

5.5   Targeting Signaling Pathway Molecules

5.5.1   Small Molecules Target Th17 Cells

By screening small molecule libraries, several groups have identified small molecular compounds that have an inhibitory function on RORγt and thereby interfere with Th17 cell differentiation. These small molecules have been demonstrated to suppress autoimmune inflammatory disease models [82].

5.5.1.1   Digoxin and Digoxin Derivatives

The cardiac glycoside digoxin was the first small molecule to be identified as a specific inhibitor of RORγ transcriptional activity in an insect cell-based reporter system as it does not affect the transcriptional activity of other transcription factors tested including RORα, DHR3 (drosophila orthologue for ROR family proteins), and VP16 [1]. Digoxin directly binds to RORγ at the ligand-binding domain (LBD) (Fig. 5.1d) [1, 83]. Addition of digoxin into a mouse Th17 differentiation system resulted in markedly reduced expression of IL-17A, IL-17F, IL-22, and IL-23R genes, whereas IL-21, Maf, RORα, BATF, and IRF4 gene expression was not affected. In addition, naive CD4+ T cell differentiation into Th1, Th2, or Treg lineage was not affected by digoxin. All these data indicate that digoxin selectively inhibits RORγt-mediated Th17 cell differentiation. The Th17 inhibition effect of digoxin was further tested in vivo in disease models. Digoxin was able to inhibit myelin oligodendrocyte glycoprotein (MOG) peptide-specific Th17 cell differentiation, attenuate EAE [1, 83], delay the onset of the disease, and reduce the severity in CIA [84, 85]. Despite the high specificity in targeting RORγt to suppress Th17 cell differentiation and efficacy in treating autoimmune inflammatory disease models, it is unlikely that digoxin will be used to treat human inflammatory conditions because of its toxicity to human cells at the high dose [1]. In a recent study, digoxin was able to inhibit induction of experimental autoimmune uveitis in mice but causes severe retinal degeneration [86]. The dose required to be therapeutic for inflammatory disease models is greater by two orders of magnitude than that used in humans for treating heart failure [87]. Application of these digoxin derivatives in human autoimmune inflammatory diseases requires further investigations. However, if such a high dose as used in mice is required for treating inflammatory diseases in humans, it is obviously not safe. The synthetic derivatives 20,22-dihydrodigoxin-21,23-diol and digoxin-21-salicylidene can specifically inhibit Th17 cell differentiation but are nontoxic to human cells in vitro [1]. Nevertheless, these data indicate that derivatives of digoxin might be used as chemical templates for the development of therapeutic agents that target RORγt and attenuate inflammatory Th17 cell function and autoimmune diseases in humans.

5.5.1.2   Other Small Molecules with Activity in Inhibition of RORγt

By screening a small chemical library, Xu et al. found that ursolic acid, a natural carboxylic acid ubiquitously present in plants, executes strong and selective inhibition of RORγt activity without affecting RORα, which led to reduced IL-17A and IL-17F expression and impaired Th17 cell differentiation [88]. Administration of ursolic acid significantly ameliorated EAE and CIA [88, 89]. Using quantitative high-throughput screening, Huh and colleagues found that diphenylpropanamide 4n among over 300,000 compounds selectively inhibited transcriptional activity of RORγt but not RORα in cells and suppressed human Th17 cell differentiation at sub-micromolar concentrations [90]. Using a similar approach, an orally efficacious RORγ inhibitor was also identified [91].

Using the liver X receptor (LXR) agonist T0901317 scaffold as a lead compound, Solt et al. [92] developed a derivative SR1001, which is able to suppress the transcriptional activity of RORα and RORγ but has no LXR activity [93]. SR1001 binds specifically to the LBD of RORα and RORγ to induce a conformational change within the LBD. SR1001 inhibited the development of murine Th17 cells and production of Th17 cytokines and effectively reduced severity of EAE in mice [93]. SR2211 is a derivative of SR1001. Unlike SR1001, SR2211 can specifically inhibit the transcriptional activity of RORγ but has no effect on RORα. SR2211 suppressed inflammatory T cell function and Th17 cell differentiation and markedly reduced joint inflammation in mice with CIA [94, 95].

5.5.1.3   TM920, TMP778, and GSK805

Xiao et al. screened a proprietary small molecule library and found several compounds binding to RORγt [96]. TM920 and TM778 were identified as highly potent and selective RORγt inhibitors [96, 97]. Both TM920 and TM778 suppressed Th17 development and inhibited IL-17 production from in vitro-differentiated Th17 cells, but TMP778 is more specific and potent and is able to block nearly all Th17 signature gene expression and has no effect on any of the other 24 nuclear receptors tested, including RORα and RORβ [96, 97]. TMP778 also potently impaired IL-17 production by human CD8+Tc17 cells, memory CD4+ T cells, and skin mononuclear cells of psoriasis patients [97]. It is noteworthy that it requires a high dose of TMP778 to exert its RORγt inhibition effect in vivo. This may potentially limit its use clinically. GSK805 is proven to be more potent than TM778 and can be orally administered. GSK805 efficiently ameliorated the severity of EAE and strongly inhibited Th17 cell differentiation in the central nervous system [96, 98].

These small molecules including digoxin are in fact not RORγt antagonists but rather inverse agonists. That is, they bind to RORγt at the LBD and diminish instead of promoting Th17 cell differentiation via interaction with other nuclear transcripters. For instance, SR1001 suppresses coactivator SRC2 binding to RORα and RORγ at the *Il17a* promoter and increases recruitment of the corepressor NCoR [93]. TMP778 and GSK805 were able to induce RORγt binding to GATA3 and led to an increase of GATA3 mRNA and protein expression. The apparent transactivation of GATA3 by RORγt may partly explain the inhibition of Th17 cell signature gene expression by TMP778 or GSK805 [96]. More recently, it has been demonstrated that TMP778 repressed more than 30 genes related to SMAD3 – a transcription factor involved in Th17 cell differentiation [98].

5.5.1.4   Small Molecules Targeting ROR in Clinical Studies

The LBD is present in both RORγt and RORγ. RORγ is widely expressed in nonimmune tissue including the heart, kidney, liver, lung, brain, and muscle. The action of these inverse agonists on RORγ may incur unwanted adverse effects in human and may limit their development as therapeutics in human. Clinical studies are required to verify. The first Phase I clinical trial of an RORγ inverse agonist has completed although the results are not yet available. This clinical trial tested the safety and efficacy of topical application of another RORγ inverse agonist GSK2981278 (https://www.clinicaltrials.gov/NCT02548052) in 15 patients with mild-to-moderate plaque psoriasis. It is expected that the consequence of effects of GSK2981278 on RORγ in nonimmune tissue is to be reported. Nonetheless, in an ex vivo assay, GSK2981278 was able to suppress IL-17A and IL-17F production for psoriatic skin, which was biopsied and cultured in the presence of GSK2981278 [99]. A small molecule RORγt reverse agonist VTP-43472 has been shown to be effective in treating moderate-to-severe psoriasis in a Phase IIa clinical trial, and a Phase IIb trial is planned [100, 101]. JTE-151 is another small molecule of the RORγt reverse agonist, which has entered a Phase I clinical trial [100].

5.5.1.5   Small Interference RNA Targeting Th17 Cells

RNA interference (RNAi) technology provides a promise for developing potential gene-specific targeted therapeutics in T cells. However, efficient delivery of small interference RNA (siRNA) into primary T cells remains a major hurdle of siRNA-based therapy [102]. Primary T cells are known to be difficult to transfect. Several methods have been developed to overcome the difficulty. Electroporation and nucleofection can deliver siRNA into T cells but they cause excessive cell death and are not suitable for in vivo use [103,104]. Chemically modified synthetic siRNA with Acell agents are not efficient in delivery [105]. Retroviral vectors can effectively infect and enter T cells. However, danger of malignant transformation limits the viral vectors to be used in vivo [102]. Nanoparticles are effective for delivering siRNA into T cells, but the delivery is not T cell specific [106]. A cell-target antibody fragment conjugated to a highly positive charged protamine peptide that binds nucleic acids has been reported for cell-specific siRNA transfection of immune cells [107, 108]. siRNAs delivered with this method can silence gene expression in cells, both in vitro and in tissues. This approach has been shown to effectively inhibit human immunodeficiency virus (HIV) infection in humanized mice [109].

Recently, aptamers have been explored to deliver siRNA into cells for therapeutic development. Aptamers are short single-stranded oligonucleotides (RNA or DNA) that can be selected from a large pool ($>1\times10^{14}$) of single-stranded oligonucleotides with random sequences [110, 111] to bind any given ligand with high specificity and high affinity. Therefore, aptamers have been referred to as "chemical antibodies." Aptamers are generally non- or low immunogenic and less expressive to generate in a large scale for clinical use. An aptamer against vascular endothelial factor has been approved by the US FDA to treat age-related macular degeneration [112]. Currently several aptamers are undergoing clinical trials [113–115]. For example, an RNA aptamer (Spiegelmer) inhibiting C-C chemokine ligand 2 (CCL2) or monocyte chemoattractant protein 1 (MCP-1) has been trialed to treat complications of type II diabetes (NCT01547897); and pegnivacogin, an aptamer inhibiting coagulation factor IXa, showed beneficial effects in suppressing ischemic events and thrombotic complications in patients with acute coronary syndrome undergoing percutaneous coronary intervention

(NCT00932100). Similar to antibodies, aptamers gain entrance to target cells via receptor-mediated endocytosis upon binding to cell surface ligands [116, 117]. Therefore, aptamers are used as a vehicle for transfer of drugs including oligonucleotides into cells. siRNA can be linked to aptamers in several ways [118]. Aptamer–siRNA chimera has been developed and tested in tumor models [119, 120] and HIV-infected human CD4+ T cells in humanized mice [121, 122].

Using CD4 aptamers T helper cell-specific delivering vehicles to deliver small hairpin RNA (shRNA) targeting RORγt has been attempted. CD4 aptamer and shRNA against RORγt were linked with a short loop sequence to form a chimera (Fig. 5.1e) [2]. CD4 aptamer binds to CD4 and carries RORγt shRNA into Th17 cells. The shRNA is processed by the cell intrinsic Dicer system to release the antisense strand. CD4 aptamer–RORγt–shRNA chimera significantly and specifically diminished RORγt expression and displayed a concentration-dependent inhibition of IL-17 A production and Th17 cell differentiation [2]. Aptamers against other cell surface proteins such as activation-induced expression CD30 by T cells are also potentially useful for delivery of siRNA/shRNA to target Th17 cells. In vivo studies are required to verify the application of this approach in disease models.

MicroRNAs (miRNAs) are small noncoding RNAs that are now recognized as essential regulators of gene expression and have been implicated in the pathogenesis of inflammatory diseases [123, 124]. Many miRNAs regulate development of Th17 cells and IL-17 cytokine function positively and negatively [125]. Manipulation of these miRNAs has therapeutic potential, for instance, inhibition of miR-155- and miR-326-reduced severity of EAE with reduction of Th17 cells [126–128]. miRNA-based therapeutics is an area of active research for development of novel therapies for cancer. Several clinical studies are undergoing for cancer therapy [129, 130]. The strategies involve delivery of miRNA or manipulation of miRNA. Similar to the application of siRNA/shRNA for clinical use, delivery of an efficient amount of miRNA is the major hurdle. Aptamer-mediated delivery is also under active investigation [129, 130].

5.5.2   Act1 Inhibition

The adaptor protein, Act1, is critical for IL-17–IL-17RA/RC signaling [131, 132]. Studies using gene knockout mice proved that Act1 is required for development of several IL-17-mediated inflammatory disease models including CIA [133], imiquimod-induced psoriasis [134], EAE and dextran sodium sulfate-induced colitis [135], cuprizone-induced demyelination [136], lupus nephritis [137], and IL-25 (IL-17E)-induced asthma [138]. All these data suggest that Act1 is a target for blocking IL-17-mediated effects in effector cells. For its intracellular location, small molecules and RNAi-based agents are the best choice to develop for targeting Act1 activity. Recently, Liu et al. found that a cell-permeable peptide, a decoy CC' loop of the Act1 SEFIR domain, is able to ameliorate IL-17 A- and IL-25-induced lung inflammation [139]. These findings suggest that the CC' loop of the Act1 SEFIR domain is a promising target for therapeutic strategies against inflammatory diseases associated with IL-17 and IL-25 signaling (see Fig. 1.2). As all IL-17Rs contain the SEFIR domain and IL-17RA is a common receptor – a component of the heterodimeric functional receptor complex for IL-17A, IL-17F, IL-17C, and IL-17E – an inhibitor to block a particular IL-17 cytokine will need to be specific to the cognate receptor chain. For example, to block IL-17E (IL-25) signaling, an inhibitor needs to specifically interfere with interaction between SEFIR of Act1 and SEFIR of IL-17RB.

5.6   Safety in Blocking IL-17/Th17 Pathway as Therapies for Inflammatory Diseases

5.6.1   Safety

In general, blocking the IL-17/Th17 pathway has been proven to be a safe modality in treating various inflammatory diseases. The safety profile in blocking upper stream cytokines including those blocking TNF, IL-1, and IL-6 is generally acceptable. The safety profile of specifically blocking IL-23 and IL-17 cytokines is similar to those of blocking other cytokines. Specifically, using ustekinumab to block IL-12/IL-23 p40 has been in the market for over 4 years and has acceptable adverse effects. The major adverse effects for these cytokine blocking agents are increased frequency of infections. It is somewhat surprising that blocking the IL-17/Th17 pathway displays no significant increase of serious infections given the importance of these cytokines in host defense. The review of safety data here will focus on fungal infection, and use secukinumab as an example to illustrate the impact of blocking the IL-17 pathway on host defenses against fungal infections as secukinumab has been exposed to the largest number of patients and long-term observation is available. The safety database covers 3430 psoriasis patients who were treated with secukinumab covering 2725 patient-years of exposure. Secukinumab was comparable to etanercept in total adverse effects. The most common adverse effects are upper respiratory infections, which are nonserious. The incidence of *Candida* infections was more frequent in a higher dose (300 mg) [140].

Candida infections include oral, vulvovaginal, cutaneous, esophageal, oropharyngeal, and genital candidiasis which are not serious and required standard antifungal therapy (Table 5.2).

It is noteworthy that therapeutic blocking of IL-17 cytokine activities in these inflammatory diseases did not reproduce the severity of clinical phenotypes seen in patients with genetic defects in the IL-17/Th17 pathway. It is reassuring that blockade of the IL-17/Th17 pathway for therapy is acceptable in clinical practice.

5.6.2   Dichotomous Effects on Crohn's Disease by Blocking IL-23 Versus IL-17 Signaling

Several lines of evidence support the pathogenic role of IL-23 and IL-17 cytokines in inflammatory bowel disease, such as Crohn's disease. Ustekinumab is efficacious in treating human Crohn's disease [27, 28]. Surprisingly, clinical trials with anti-IL-17A or anti-IL-17RA show either no improvement or even

TABLE 5.2 Incidence of candidiasis in patients with psoriasis treated with secukinumab[a]

Incidence rate of candidiasis	Secukinumab (300 mg)	Secukinumab (150 mg)	Etanercept	Placebo
12 weeks	1.2	0.4	0.3	0.3
52 weeks	3.55	1.85	1.0	1.35

[a]Pooled data from a total of 3430 patients with psoriasis from all clinical trials. Incidence rate is expressed as rate per 100 patient-years

exacerbation of Crohn's disease [55, 141]. These findings appear paradoxical given the fact that elevated levels of both IL-23 and IL-17 are detected in Crohn's disease and in mouse models of colitis. However, observations from recent animal models of colitis provide an explanation. In dextran sodium sulfate-induced colitis, anti-IL-17A antibody treatment or IL-17A knocked out exacerbated the disease [57, 58, 142]. In colitis, the dominant function of IL-17 may be to preserve the intestinal epithelial barrier [143, 144]. IL-17A is able to stimulate gut epithelial cell proliferation and healing in cooperation with fibroblast growth factor receptor [142]. It appears that the protective IL-17A is derived from γδT cells. The production of IL-17A by these γδT cells is independent of IL-23 [143]. In addition, abrogation of IL-17RA in the enteric epithelium leads to the commensal dysbiosis of gut microbiome and increased serum granulocyte macrophage-colony stimulator factor (GM-CSF) [145].

References

1. Fujita-Sato S, Ito S, Isobe T, et al. Structural basis of digoxin that antagonizes RORgamma t receptor activity and suppresses Th17 cell differentiation and interleukin (IL)-17 production. J Biol Chem. 2011;286:31409–17.
2. Song P, Chou YK, Zhang X, et al. CD4 aptamer-RORgammat shRNA chimera inhibits IL-17 synthesis by human CD4(+) T cells. Biochem Biophys Res Commun. 2014;452:1040–5.
3. Zheng Y, Sun L, Jiang T, Zhang D, He D, Nie H. TNFalpha promotes Th17 cell differentiation through IL-6 and IL-1beta produced by monocytes in rheumatoid arthritis. J Immunol Res. 2014;2014:385352.
4. Piaserico S, Sandini E, Saldan A, Abate D. Effects of TNF-alpha inhibitors on circulating Th17 cells in patients affected by severe psoriasis. Drug Dev Res. 2014;75(Suppl 1):S73–6.
5. Chen DY, Chen YM, Chen HH, Hsieh CW, Lin CC, Lan JL. Increasing levels of circulating Th17 cells and interleukin-17 in rheumatoid arthritis patients with an inadequate response to anti-TNF-alpha therapy. Arthritis Res Ther. 2011; 13:R126.

6. Alzabin S, Abraham SM, Taher TE, et al. Incomplete response of inflammatory arthritis to TNFalpha blockade is associated with the Th17 pathway. Ann Rheum Dis. 2012;71:1741–8.

7. Hull N, Williams RO, Pathan E, Alzabin S, Abraham S, Taylor PC. Anti-tumour necrosis factor treatment increases circulating T helper type 17 cells similarly in different types of inflammatory arthritis. Clin Exp Immunol. 2015;181:401–6.

8. Xueyi L, Lina C, Zhenbiao W, Qing H, Qiang L, Zhu P. Levels of circulating Th17 cells and regulatory T cells in ankylosing spondylitis patients with an inadequate response to anti-TNF-alpha therapy. J Clin Immunol. 2013;33:151–61.

9. Komatsu N, Okamoto K, Sawa S, et al. Pathogenic conversion of Foxp3+ T cells into TH17 cells in autoimmune arthritis. Nat Med. 2014;20:62–8.

10. Guggino G, Giardina AR, Raimondo S, Giardina G, et al. Targeting IL-6 signalling in early rheumatoid arthritis is followed by Th1 and Th17 suppression and Th2 expansion. Clin Exp Rheumatol. 2014;32:77–81.

11. Samson M, Audia S, Janikashvili N, et al. Brief report: inhibition of interleukin-6 function corrects Th17/Treg cell imbalance in patients with rheumatoid arthritis. Arthritis Rheumatol. 2012;64:2499–503.

12. Sieper J, Porter-Brown B, Thompson L, Harari O, Dougados M. Assessment of short-term symptomatic efficacy of tocilizumab in ankylosing spondylitis: results of randomised, placebo-controlled trials. Ann Rheum Dis. 2014;73:95–100.

13. Sieper J, Braun J, Kay J, et al. Sarilumab for the treatment of ankylosing spondylitis: results of a Phase II, randomised, double-blind, placebo-controlled study (ALIGN). Ann Rheum Dis. 2015;74:1051–7.

14. Mease P, Gottlieb SB, Berman A, et al. The efficacy and safety of clazakizumab, an anti-interleukin-6 monoclonal antibody, in a Phase 2b study of adults with active psoriatic arthritis. Arthritis Rheum. 2016;68:2163–73.

15. Yang XO, Panopoulos AD, Nurieva R, et al. STAT3 regulates cytokine-mediated generation of inflammatory helper T cells. J Biol Chem. 2007;282:9358–63.

16. McKeage K. Ustekinumab: a review of its use in psoriatic arthritis. Drugs. 2014;74:1029–39.

17. Leonardi CL, Kimball AB, Papp KA, et al. Efficacy and safety of ustekinumab, a human interleukin-12/23 monoclonal antibody, in patients with psoriasis: 76-week results from a randomised,

double-blind, placebo-controlled trial (PHOENIX 1). Lancet. 2008;371:1665–74.

18. Papp KA, Langley RG, Lebwohl M, et al. Efficacy and safety of ustekinumab, a human interleukin-12/23 monoclonal antibody, in patients with psoriasis: 52-week results from a randomised, double-blind, placebo-controlled trial (PHOENIX 2). Lancet. 2008;371:1675–84.

19. Griffiths CE, Strober BE, van de Kerkhof P, et al. Comparison of ustekinumab and etanercept for moderate-to-severe psoriasis. N Engl J Med. 2010;362:118–28.

20. McInnes IB, Kavanaugh A, Gottlieb AB, et al. Efficacy and safety of ustekinumab in patients with active psoriatic arthritis: 1 year results of the phase 3, multicentre, double-blind, placebo-controlled PSUMMIT 1 trial. Lancet. 2013;382:780–9.

21. Ritchlin C, Rahman P, Kavanaugh A, et al. Efficacy and safety of the anti-IL-12/23 p40 monoclonal antibody, ustekinumab, in patients with active psoriatic arthritis despite conventional non-biological and biological anti-tumour necrosis factor therapy: 6-month and 1-year results of the phase 3, multicentre, double-blind, placebo-controlled, randomised PSUMMIT 2 trial. Ann Rheum Dis. 2014;73:990–9.

22. Papp KA, Griffiths CE, Gordon K, et al. Reich, Long-term safety of ustekinumab in patients with moderate-to-severe psoriasis: final results from 5 years of follow-up. Br J Dermatol. 2013;168:844–54.

23. Sorenson E, Koo J. Evidence-based adverse effects of biologic agents in the treatment of moderate-to-severe psoriasis: Providing clarity to an opaque topic. J Dermatolog Treat. 2015;26:493–501.

24. Papp K, Gottlieb AB, Naldi L, et al. Safety Surveillance for Ustekinumab and Other Psoriasis Treatments From the Psoriasis Longitudinal Assessment and Registry (PSOLAR). J Drugs Dermatol. 2015;14:706–14.

25. Warren RB, Smith CH, Yiu ZZ, et al. Differential drug survival of biologic therapies for the treatment of psoriasis: a prospective observational cohort study from the British Association of Dermatologists Biologic Interventions Register (BADBIR). J Invest Dermatol. 2015;135:2632–40.

26. Gniadecki R, Bang B, Bryld LE, Iversen L, Lasthein S, Skov L. Comparison of long-term drug survival and safety of biologic agents in patients with psoriasis vulgaris. Br J Dermatol. 2015;172:244–52.

27. Sandborn WJ, Feagan BG, Fedorak RN, et al. A randomized trial of Ustekinumab, a human interleukin-12/23 monoclonal antibody, in patients with moderate-to-severe Crohn's disease. Gastroenterology. 2008;135:1130–41.

28. Sandborn WJ, Gasink C, Gao LL, et al. Ustekinumab induction and maintenance therapy in refractory Crohn's disease. N Engl J Med. 2012;367:1519–28.

29. Levin AA, Gottlieb AB. Specific targeting of interleukin-23p19 as effective treatment for psoriasis. J Am Acad Dermatol. 2014;70:555–61.

30. Hoeve MA, Savage ND, de Boer T, et al. Divergent effects of IL-12 and IL-23 on the production of IL-17 by human T cells. Eur J Immunol. 2006;36:661–70.

31. Segal BM, Constantinescu CS, Raychaudhuri A, Kim L, Fidelus-Gort R, Kasper LH. Repeated subcutaneous injections of IL12/23 p40 neutralising antibody, ustekinumab, in patients with relapsing-remitting multiple sclerosis: a phase II, double-blind, placebo-controlled, randomised, dose-ranging study. Lancet Neurol. 2008;7:796–804.

32. Campa M, Mansouri B, Warren R, Menter A. A review of biologic therapies targeting IL-23 and IL-17 for use in moderate-to-severe plaque psoriasis. Dermatol Ther (Heidelb). 2016;6:1–12.

33. Gordon KB, Langley RG, Gottlieb AB, et al. A phase III, randomized, controlled trial of the fully human IL-12/23 mAb briakinumab in moderate-to-severe psoriasis. J Invest Dermatol. 2012;132:304–14.

34. Panaccione R, Sandborn WJ, Gordon GL, et al. Briakinumab for treatment of Crohn's disease: results of a randomized trial. Inflamm Bowel Dis. 2015;21:1329–40.

35. Khanna R, Preiss JC, MacDonald JK, Timmer A. Anti-IL-12/23p40 antibodies for induction of remission in Crohn's disease. Cochrane Database Syst Rev. 2015;5:CD007572.

36. Reich K, Langley RG, Papp KA, et al. A 52-week trial comparing briakinumab with methotrexate in patients with psoriasis. N Engl J Med. 2011;365:1586–96.

37. Yeremenko N, Paramarta JE, Baeten D. The interleukin-23/interleukin-17 immune axis as a promising new target in the treatment of spondyloarthritis. Curr Opin Rheumatol. 2014;26:361–70.

38. Papp K, Thaci D, Reich K, et al. Tildrakizumab (MK-3222), an anti-interleukin-23p19 monoclonal antibody, improves psoriasis in a phase IIb randomized placebo-controlled trial. Br J Dermatol. 2015;173:930–9.

39. Kopp T, Riedl E, Bangert C, et al. Clinical improvement in psoriasis with specific targeting of interleukin-23. Nature. 2015;521:222–6.

40. Krueger JG, Ferris LK, Menter A, et al. Anti-IL-23 A mAb BI 655066 for treatment of moderate-to-severe psoriasis: Safety, efficacy, pharmacokinetics, and biomarker results of a single-rising-dose, randomized, double-blind, placebo-controlled trial. J Allergy Clin Immunol. 2015;136:116–24. e7

41. Gordon KB, Duffin KC, Bissonnette R, et al. A Phase 2 trial of guselkumab versus adalimumab for plaque psoriasis. N Engl J Med. 2015;373:136–44.

42. Sofen H, Smith S, Matheson RT, et al. Guselkumab (an IL-23-specific mAb) demonstrates clinical and molecular response in patients with moderate-to-severe psoriasis. J Allergy Clin Immunol. 2014;133:1032–40.

43. Langley RG, Elewski BE, Lebwohl M, et al. Secukinumab in plaque psoriasis--results of two phase 3 trials. N Engl J Med. 2014;371:326–38.

44. Hueber W, Patel DD, Dryja T, et al. Effects of AIN457, a fully human antibody to interleukin-17 A, on psoriasis, rheumatoid arthritis, and uveitis. Sci Transl Med. 2010;2:52ra72.

45. Langley RG, Feldman SR, Nyirady J, van de Kerkhof P, Papavassilis C. The 5-point Investigator's Global Assessment (IGA) Scale: A modified tool for evaluating plaque psoriasis severity in clinical trials. J Dermatolog Treat. 2015;26:23–31.

46. Blauvelt A, Prinz JC, Gottlieb AB, et al. Secukinumab administration by pre-filled syringe: efficacy, safety and usability results from a randomized controlled trial in psoriasis (FEATURE). Br J Dermatol. 2015;172:484–93.

47. Paul C, Lacour JP, Tedremets L, et al. Efficacy, safety and usability of secukinumab administration by autoinjector/pen in psoriasis: a randomized, controlled trial (JUNCTURE). J Eur Acad Dermatol Venereol. 2015;29:1082–90.

48. Mease PJ, McInnes IB, Kirkham B, et al. Secukinumab inhibition of interleukin-17 A in patients with psoriatic arthritis. N Engl J Med. 2015;373:1329–39.

49. McInnes IB, Mease PJ, Kirkham B, et al. Secukinumab, a human anti-interleukin-17 A monoclonal antibody, in patients with psoriatic arthritis (FUTURE 2): a randomised, double-blind, placebo-controlled, phase 3 trial. Lancet. 2015;386:1137–46.

50. Baeten D, Sieper J, Braun J, et al. Secukinumab, an interleukin-17 A inhibitor, in ankylosing spondylitis. N Engl J Med. 2015;373:2534–48.

51. Genovese MC, Durez P, Richards HB, et al. Efficacy and safety of secukinumab in patients with rheumatoid arthritis: a phase II, dose-finding, double-blind, randomised, placebo controlled study. Ann Rheum Dis. 2013;72:863–9.

52. Genovese MC, Durez P, Richards HB, et al. One-year efficacy and safety results of secukinumab in patients with rheumatoid arthritis: phase II, dose-finding, double-blind, randomized, placebo-controlled study. J Rheumatol. 2014;41:414–21.

53. Tlustochowicz W, Rahman P, Seriolo B, et al. Efficacy and safety of subcutaneous and intravenous loading dose regimens of secukinumab in patients with active rheumatoid arthritis: results from a randomized Phase II study. J Rheumatol. 2016;43: 495–503.

54. Burmester GR, Durez P, Shestakova G, et al. Association of HLA-DRB1 alleles with clinical responses to the anti-interleukin-17 A monoclonal antibody secukinumab in active rheumatoid arthritis. Rheumatology (Oxford). 2016;55:49–55.

55. Hueber W, Sands BE, Lewitzky S, et al. Secukinumab, a human anti-IL-17 A monoclonal antibody, for moderate to severe Crohn's disease: unexpected results of a randomised, double-blind placebo-controlled trial. Gut. 2012;61:1693–700.

56. Strober W, Zhang F, Kitani A, Fuss I, Fichtner-Feigl S. Proinflammatory cytokines underlying the inflammation of Crohn's disease. Curr Opin Gastroenterol. 2010;26:310–7.

57. O'Connor Jr W, Kamanaka M, Booth CJ, et al. A protective function for interleukin 17 A in T cell-mediated intestinal inflammation. Nat Immunol. 2009;10:603–9.

58. Ogawa A, Andoh A, Araki Y, Bamba T, Fujiyama Y. Neutralization of interleukin-17 aggravates dextran sulfate sodium-induced colitis in mice. Clin Immunol. 2004;110:55–62.

59. Luchtman DW, Ellwardt E, Larochelle C, Zipp F. IL-17 and related cytokines involved in the pathology and immunotherapy of multiple sclerosis: Current and future developments. Cytokine Growth Factor Rev. 2014;25:403–13.

60. Farahnik B, Beroukhim K, Zhu TH, et al. Ixekizumab for the treatment of psoriasis: a review of Phase III trials. Dermatol Ther (Heidelb). 2016;6:25–37.

61. Griffiths CE, Reich K, Lebwohl M, et al. Comparison of ixekizumab with etanercept or placebo in moderate-to-severe psoriasis (UNCOVER-2 and UNCOVER-3): results from two phase 3 randomised trials. Lancet. 2015;386:541–51.

62. Mease PJ, van der Heijde D, Ritchlin CT, et al. A randomized, double-blind, active- and placebo-controlled Phase 3 study of

efficacy and safety of ixekizumab, adalimumab, and placebo therapy in patients naïve to biologic disease modifying antirheumatic drugs with active psoriatic arthritis. Arthritis Rheumatol. 2015;67 (suppl 10).

63. Gottlieb AB, Mease PJ, Cuchacovich RS, et al. Ixekizumab improves physical function, quality of life, and work productivity in biologic disease-modifying antirheumatic drug-naive patients with active psoriatic arthritis. Arthritis Rheumatol. 2015;67 (suppl 10).

64. Genovese MC, Van den Bosch F, Roberson SA, et al. LY2439821, a humanized anti-interleukin-17 monoclonal antibody, in the treatment of patients with rheumatoid arthritis: a phase I randomized, double-blind, placebo-controlled, proof-of-concept study. Arthritis Rheumatol. 2010;62:929–39.

65. Genovese MC, Braun DK, Erickson JS, et al. Safety and efficacy of open-label subcutaneous ixekizumab treatment for 48 weeks in a Phase II study in biologic-naive and TNF-IR patients with rheumatoid arthritis. J Rheumatol. 2016;43:289–97.

66. Genovese MC, Greenwald M, Cho CS, et al. A phase II randomized study of subcutaneous ixekizumab, an anti-interleukin-17 monoclonal antibody, in rheumatoid arthritis patients who were naive to biologic agents or had an inadequate response to tumor necrosis factor inhibitors. Arthritis Rheumatol. 2014;66:1693–704.

67. Coimbra S, Figueiredo A, Santos-Silva A. Brodalumab: an evidence-based review of its potential in the treatment of moderate-to-severe psoriasis. Core Evid. 2014;9:89–97.

68. Russell CB, Rand H, Bigler J, et al. Gene expression profiles normalized in psoriatic skin by treatment with brodalumab, a human anti-IL-17 receptor monoclonal antibody. J Immunol. 2014;192:3828–36.

69. Papp KA, Leonardi C, Menter A, et al. Brodalumab, an anti-interleukin-17-receptor antibody for psoriasis. N Engl J Med. 2012;366:1181–9.

70. Papp K, Reich K, Leonardi C, et al. Efficacy and safety of brodalumab in patients with moderate to severe plaque psoriasis: Results of AMAGINE-1, a phase 3, randomized, double-blind, placebo-controlled study through week 12. J Am Acad Dermatol. 2015;72:AB233.

71. Lebwohl M, Strober B, Menter A, et al. Phase 3 studies comparing brodalumab with ustekinumab in psoriasis. N Engl J Med. 2015;373:1318–28.

72. Mease PJ, Genovese MC, Greenwald MW, et al. Brodalumab, an anti-IL17RA monoclonal antibody, in psoriatic arthritis. N Engl J Med. 2014;370:2295–306.

73. Genovese MC, Cohen S, Moreland L, et al. Combination therapy with etanercept and anakinra in the treatment of patients with rheumatoid arthritis who have been treated unsuccessfully with methotrexate. Arthritis Rheumatol. 2004;50:1412–9.

74. Weinblatt M, Schiff M, Goldman A, et al. Selective costimulation modulation using abatacept in patients with active rheumatoid arthritis while receiving etanercept: a randomised clinical trial. Ann Rheum Dis. 2007;66:228–34.

75. Fischer JA, Hueber AJ, Wilson S, et al. Combined inhibition of tumor necrosis factor alpha and interleukin-17 as a therapeutic opportunity in rheumatoid arthritis: development and characterization of a novel bispecific antibody. Arthritis Rheumatol. 2015;67:51–62.

76. Spiess C, Zhai Q, Carter PJ. Alternative molecular formats and therapeutic applications for bispecific antibodies. Mol Immunol. 2015;67:95–106.

77. Fleischmann R, Wagner F, Kivitz AJ, et al. Safety, tolerability, and pharcodynamics of ABT-122, a dual TNF- and IL-17-targeted dural variable domain (DVD)-IgTM in subjects with rheumatoid arthritis. Arthritis Rheumatol. 2015;67:1262–3.

78. Glatt S, Helmer E, Strimenopoulou F, et al. First-in-human IL-17 A and IL-17F blockade with bimekizumab in patients with mild-to-moderate psoriasis: results of a randomized, placebo-controlled, single-dose-escalating study. 74th Annual Meeting of American Academy of Dermatology, Wanshington DC, March 4–6, 2016.

79. Patel DD, Kuchroo VK. Th17 Cell Pathway in Human Immunity: Lessons from Genetics and Therapeutic Interventions. Immunity. 2015;43:1040–51.

80. Silacci M, Lembke W, Woods R, et al. Discovery and characterization of COVA322, a clinical-stage bispecific TNF/IL-17 A inhibitor for the treatment of inflammatory diseases. MAbs. 2016;8:141–9.

81. Nunez-Prado N, Compte M, Harwood S, et al. The coming of age of engineered multivalent antibodies. Drug Discov Today. 2015;20:588–94.

82. Lin H, Song P, Zhao Y, et al. Targeting Th17 cells with small molecules and small interference RNA. Mediators Inflamm. 2015;2015:290657.

83. Huh JR, Leung MW, Huang P, et al. Digoxin and its derivatives suppress TH17 cell differentiation by antagonizing RORgammat activity. Nature. 2011;472:486–90.

84. Lee J, Baek S, Lee DG, et al. Digoxin ameliorates autoimmune arthritis via suppression of Th17 differentiation. Int Immunopharmacol. 2015;26:103–11.

85. Cascao R, Vidal B, Raquel H, et al. Effective treatment of rat adjuvant-induced arthritis by celastrol. Autoimmun Rev. 2012;11:856–62.

86. Hinshaw SJ, Ogbeifun O, Wandu WS, et al. Digoxin inhibits induction of experimental autoimmune uveitis in mice, but causes severe retinal degeneration. Invest Ophthalmol Vis Sci. 2016;57:1441–7.

87. Kanji S, MacLean RD. Cardiac glycoside toxicity: more than 200 years and counting. Crit Care Clin. 2012;28:527–35.

88. Xu T, Wang X, Zhong B, Nurieva RI, Ding S, Dong C. Ursolic acid suppresses interleukin-17 (IL-17) production by selectively antagonizing the function of RORgamma t protein. J Biol Chem. 2011;286:22707–10.

89. Baek SY, Lee J, Lee DG, et al. Ursolic acid ameliorates autoimmune arthritis via suppression of Th17 and B cell differentiation. Acta Pharmacol Sin. 2014;35:1177–87.

90. Huh JR, Englund EE, Wang H, et al. Identification of potent and selective diphenylpropanamide RORgamma inhibitors. ACS Med Chem Lett. 2013;4:79–84.

91. Hirata K, Kotoku M, Seki N, et al. SAR Exploration guided by LE and Fsp(3): discovery of a selective and orally efficacious RORgamma inhibitor. ACS Med Chem Lett. 2016;7:23–7.

92. Kumar N, Solt LA, Conkright JJ, et al. The benzenesulfoamide T0901317 [N-(2,2,2-trifluoroethyl)-N-[4-[2,2,2-trifluoro-1-hydroxy-1-(trifluoromethyl)ethy l]phenyl]-benzenesulfonamide] is a novel retinoic acid receptor-related orphan receptor-alpha/gamma inverse agonist. Mol Pharmacol. 2010;77:228–36.

93. Solt LA, Kumar N, Nuhant P, et al. Suppression of TH17 differentiation and autoimmunity by a synthetic ROR ligand. Nature. 2011;472:491–4.

94. Chang MR, Lyda B, Kamenecka TM, Griffin PR. Pharmacologic repression of retinoic acid receptor-related orphan nuclear receptor gamma is therapeutic in the collagen-induced arthritis experimental model. Arthritis Rheumatol. 2014;66:579–88.

95. Kumar N, Lyda B, Chang MR, et al. Identification of SR2211: a potent synthetic RORgamma-selective modulator. ACS Chem Biol. 2012;7:672–7.

96. Xiao S, Yosef N, Yang J, et al. Small-molecule RORgammat antagonists inhibit T helper 17 cell transcriptional network by divergent mechanisms. Immunity. 2014;40:477–89.

97. Skepner J, Ramesh R, Trocha M, et al. Pharmacologic inhibition of RORgammat regulates Th17 signature gene expression and suppresses cutaneous inflammation in vivo. J Immunol. 2014;192:2564–75.

98. Skepner J, Trocha M, Ramesh R, et al. In vivo regulation of gene expression and T helper type 17 differentiation by RORgammat inverse agonists. Immunology. 2015;145:347–56.

99. Smith SH, Peredo CE, Takeda Y, et al. Development of a topical treatment for psoriasis targeting RORgamma: from bench to skin. PLoS ONE. 2016;11:2016. e0147979

100. Gege C. Retinoid-related orphan receptor gamma t (RORgammat) inhibitors from Vitae Pharmaceuticals (WO2015116904) and structure proposal for their Phase I candidate VTP-43742. Expert Opin Ther Pat. 2016;26:1–8.

101. Vitae Pharmaceuticals. Autoimmune diseases. http://vitaepharma.com/pipeline/autoimmune-diseases/. Accessed 12 Aug 2016.

102. Freeley M, Long A. Advances in siRNA delivery to T-cells: potential clinical applications for inflammatory disease, cancer and infection. Biochem J. 2013;455:133–47.

103. Gehl J. Electroporation: theory and methods, perspectives for drug delivery, gene therapy and research. Acta Physiol Scand. 2003;177:437–47.

104. Lai W, Chang CH, Farber DL. Gene transfection and expression in resting and activated murine CD4 T cell subsets. J Immunol Methods. 2003;282:93–102.

105. Gomez-Valades AG, Llamas M, Blanch S, et al. Specific Jak3 downregulation in lymphocytes impairs gammac cytokine signal transduction and alleviates antigen-driven inflammation in vivo. Mol Ther Nucleic Acids. 2012;1:e42.

106. Liu Z, Winters M, Holodniy M, Dai H. siRNA delivery into human T cells and primary cells with carbon-nanotube transporters. Angew Chem Int Ed Engl. 2007;46:2023–7.

107. Song E, Zhu P, Lee SK, et al. Antibody mediated in vivo delivery of small interfering RNAs via cell-surface receptors. Nat Biotechnol. 2005;23:709–17.

108. Peer D, Zhu P, Carman CV, Lieberman J, Shimaoka M. Selective gene silencing in activated leukocytes by targeting siRNAs to the integrin lymphocyte function-associated antigen-1. Proc Natl Acad Sci U S A. 2007;104:4095–100.

109. Kumar P, Ban HS, Kim SS, et al. T cell-specific siRNA delivery suppresses HIV-1 infection in humanized mice. Cell. 2008;134:577–86.

110. Cerchia L, de Franciscis V. Targeting cancer cells with nucleic acid aptamers. Trends Biotechnol. 2010;28:517–25.

111. Keefe AD, Szostak JW. Functional proteins from a random-sequence library. Nature. 2001;410:715–8.

112. Ng EW, Adamis AP. Anti-VEGF aptamer (pegaptanib) therapy for ocular vascular diseases. Ann N Y Acad Sci. 2006;1082: 151–71.

113. Keefe AD, Pai S, Ellington A. Aptamers as therapeutics. Nat Rev Drug Discov. 2010;9:537–50.

114. Burnett JC, Rossi JJ. RNA-based therapeutics: current progress and future prospects. Chem Biol. 2012;19:60–71.

115. Sundaram P, Kurniawan H, Byrne ME, Wower J. Therapeutic RNA aptamers in clinical trials. Eur J Pharm Sci. 2013;48: 259–71.

116. Bruno JG. A review of therapeutic aptamer conjugates with emphasis on new approaches. Pharmaceuticals (Basel). 2013;6: 340–57.

117. Meng L, Yang L, Zhao X, et al. Targeted delivery of chemotherapy agents using a liver cancer-specific aptamer. PLoS One. 2012;7:e33434.

118. Dassie JP, Giangrande PH. Current progress on aptamer-targeted oligonucleotide therapeutics. Ther Deliv. 2013;4:1527–46.

119. Dassie JP, Liu XY, Thomas GS, et al. Systemic administration of optimized aptamer-siRNA chimeras promotes regression of PSMA-expressing tumors. Nat Biotechnol. 2009;27:839–49.

120. McNamara 2nd JO, Andrechek ER, Wang Y, et al. Cell type-specific delivery of siRNAs with aptamer-siRNA chimeras. Nat Biotechnol. 2006;24:1005–15.

121. Wheeler LA, Trifonova R, Vrbanac V, et al. Inhibition of HIV transmission in human cervicovaginal explants and humanized mice using CD4 aptamer-siRNA chimeras. J Clin Invest. 2011;121:2401–12.

122. Wheeler LA, Vrbanac V, Trifonova R, et al. Durable knockdown and protection from HIV transmission in humanized mice treated with gel-formulated CD4 aptamer-siRNA chimeras. Mol Ther. 2013;21:1378–89.

123. Carthew RW, Sontheimer EJ. Origins and Mechanisms of miRNAs and siRNAs. Cell. 2009;136:642–55.

124. Garo LP, Murugaiyan G. Contribution of MicroRNAs to autoimmune diseases. Cell Mol Life Sci. 2016;73:2041–51.

125. Khan D, Ansar AS. Regulation of IL-17 in autoimmune diseases by transcription factors and microRNAs. Front Genet. 2015;6:236.

126. Zhang J, Cheng Y, Cui W, Li M, Li B, Guo L. MicroRNA-155 modulates Th1 and Th17 cell differentiation and is associated with multiple sclerosis and experimental autoimmune encephalomyelitis. J Neuroimmunol. 2014;266:56–63.
127. Murugaiyan G, Beynon V, Mittal A, Joller N, Weiner HL. Silencing microRNA-155 ameliorates experimental autoimmune encephalomyelitis. J Immunol. 2011;187:2213–21.
128. Du C, Liu C, Kang J, et al. MicroRNA miR-326 regulates TH-17 differentiation and is associated with the pathogenesis of multiple sclerosis. Nat Immunol. 2009;10:1252–9.
129. Monroig-Bosque Pdel C, Rivera CA, Calin GA. MicroRNAs in cancer therapeutics: "from the bench to the bedside". Expert Opin Biol Ther. 2015;15:1381–5.
130. Abba ML, Patil N, Leupold JH, et al. MicroRNAs as novel targets and tools in cancer therapy. Cancer Lett. 2016; doi:10.1016/j.canlet.2016.03.043. [Epub ahead of print]
131. Gu C, Wu L, Li X. IL-17 family: cytokines, receptors and signaling. Cytokine. 2013;64:477–85.
132. Song X, Qian Y. IL-17 family cytokines mediated signaling in the pathogenesis of inflammatory diseases. Cell Signal. 2013;25:2335–47.
133. Pisitkun P, Claudio E, Ren N, Wang H, Siebenlist U. The adaptor protein CIKS/ACT1 is necessary for collagen-induced arthritis, and it contributes to the production of collagen-specific antibody. Arthritis Rheumatol. 2010;62:3334–44.
134. Ha HL, Wang H, Pisitkun P, et al. IL-17 drives psoriatic inflammation via distinct, target cell-specific mechanisms. Proc Natl Acad Sci USAmerica. 2014;111:E3422–31.
135. Qian Y, Liu C, Hartupee J, et al. The adaptor Act1 is required for interleukin 17-dependent signaling associated with autoimmune and inflammatory disease. Nat Immunol. 2007;8:247–56.
136. Kang Z, Altuntas CZ, Gulen MF, et al. Astrocyte-restricted ablation of interleukin-17-induced Act1-mediated signaling ameliorates autoimmune encephalomyelitis. Immunity. 2010;32:414–25.
137. Pisitkun P, Ha HL, Wang H, et al. Interleukin-17 cytokines are critical in development of fatal lupus glomerulonephritis. Immunity. 2012;37:1104–15.
138. Claudio E, Sonder SU, Saret S, et al. The adaptor protein CIKS/Act1 is essential for IL-25-mediated allergic airway inflammation. J Immunol. 2009;182:1617–30.

139. Liu C, Swaidani S, Qian W, et al. CC' loop decoy peptide blocks the interaction between Act1 and IL-17RA to attenuate IL-17- and IL-25-induced inflammation. Sci Signal. 2011;4:ra72.

140. US Food and Drug Administration. Secukinumab (AIN457) Advisory Committee Briefing Material. http://google2.fda.gov/search?q=secukinumab+advisory+committee+briefing+materi al&client=FDAgov&site=FDAgov&lr=&proxystylesheet=FD Agov&requiredfields=-archive%3AYes&output=xml:no_ dtd&getfields=. Accessed 12 Sep 2016.

141. Targan SR, Feagan BG, Vermeire S, et al. A randomized, double-blind, placebo-controlled study to evaluate the safety, tolerability, and efficacy of AMG 827 in subjects with moderate to severe Crohn's disease. Gastroenterology. 2012;143:e26.

142. Song X, Dai D, He X, et al. Growth factor FGF2 cooperates with interleukin-17 to repair intestinal epithelial damage. Immunity. 2015;43:488–501.

143. Lee JS, Tato CM, Joyce-Shaikh B, et al. Interleukin-23-independent IL-17 production regulates intestinal epithelial permeability. Immunity. 2015;43:727–38.

144. Maxwell JR, Zhang Y, Brown WA, et al. Differential roles for interleukin-23 and interleukin-17 in intestinal immunoregulation. Immunity. 2015;43:739–50.

145. Kumar P, Monin L, Castillo P, et al. Intestinal interleukin-17 receptor signaling mediates reciprocal control of the gut microbiota and autoimmune inflammation. Immunity. 2016;44: 659–71.

Chapter 6
Concluding Remarks

The family of IL-17 cytokines is one of the most ancient cytokines that plays an important role in host defense. In particular, IL-17 cytokines are critical for cutaneous and mucosal immunity against extracellular pathogen and fungal infections. Cells of both innate and acquired immune arms produce the IL-17 cytokine. However, aberrant production and dysregulation of IL-17 cytokine signaling has been linked to several autoimmune inflammatory diseases. Data from experiments in animal models and humans with genetic defects in the IL-17 pathway tend to suggest that IL-17 cytokines produced by innate cells are more important for host defense, while IL-17 cytokines derived from Th17 cells are associated with inflammation in autoimmune diseases. Nonetheless, therapeutic strategies applied by current global approaches, which is blocking the effector IL-17 cytokine (IL-17A and IL-17F) activity, have achieved remarkable efficacy with an acceptable safety profile. The most impressive efficacy is in treating psoriasis. This may also reflect the nonimmune effects of IL-17 cytokines on keratinocytes. Thus, IL-17A is a potent cytokine stimulating keratinocyte proliferation.

Small molecules acting as RORγt inverse agonists are effective in treating animal models of inflammatory diseases but still need to be confirmed in clinical trials. Compared with

C.-Q. Chu, *Targeting the IL-17 Pathway in Inflammatory Disorders*, DOI 10.1007/978-3-319-28040-0_6,
© Springer International Publishing Switzerland 2017

monoclonal antibodies, small molecules are less expensive to manufacture, which can be advantageous. RNAi-based therapy offers more precise targeting, but delivery is technically challenging, which will hurdle its clinical application.

Printed in the United States
By Bookmasters